ROUTLEDGE LIBRARY EDITIONS:
NURSE EDUCATION AND
NURSING CARE

Volume 20

PSYCHOLOGY FOR STUDENT NURSES

PSYCHOLOGY FOR STUDENT NURSES

JESSIE WILLIAMS

Routledge
Taylor & Francis Group
LONDON AND NEW YORK

First published in 1954 and as a second revised edition in 1957
by Methuen & Co. Ltd.

This edition first published in 2026
by Routledge
4 Park Square, Milton Park, Abingdon, Oxon OX14 4RN

and by Routledge
605 Third Avenue, New York, NY 10158

Routledge is an imprint of the Taylor & Francis Group, an informa business

British Library Cataloguing in Publication Data
A catalogue record for this book is available from the British Library

ISBN: 978-1-041-11658-5 (Set)
ISBN: 978-1-041-11631-8 (Volume 20) (hbk)
ISBN: 978-1-041-11639-4 (Volume 20) (pbk)
ISBN: 978-1-003-66089-7 (Volume 20) (ebk)

DOI: 10.4324/9781003660897

PSYCHOLOGY
FOR STUDENT NURSES

by

JESSIE WILLIAMS, M.A.

Senior Clinical Psychologist, Guy's Hospital, London. Formerly Senior Psychologist, Hospital for Sick Children, Great Ormond Street, London. Sometime Psychologist, University College Hospital, and Lecturer, University College, London

METHUEN & CO. LTD. LONDON
36 Essex Street, Strand, W.C.2

First published March 11th, 1954
Second edition (revised) 1957

2·1

CATALOGUE NO. 5700/U

PRINTED IN GREAT BRITAIN BY
BRADFORD AND DICKENS LONDON WC1
AND BOUND BY JAMES BURN AND CO LTD ESHER

AUTHOR'S NOTE

MY indebtedness to many colleagues and teachers in the field of psychology will be clear throughout this book but I should like particularly to acknowledge the debt I owe to the teachings of Susan Isaacs and to the studies of Bowlby and Burlingham and Freud to which I have referred in the text and on which I have freely drawn.

Nor can I send this small book out into the world without recording all I have gained in knowledge and experience from the Hospital for Sick Children, Great Ormond Street, London, and especially from many years' association with Dr. Mildred Creak, Physician in Psychological Medicine to this hospital. To Miss K. Biggin, Principal Sister Tutor of the hospital, I owe a debt of gratitude for many helpful discussions on the teaching of student nurses. I should also like to acknowledge my indebtedness to my colleagues at Guy's Hospital and to my former colleagues in the Department of Psychological Medicine, University College Hospital, London, and particularly to my friend Miss Grace Rawlings, to whom this book owes its beginnings.

I am grateful for permission to quote passages from *Infants Without Families*, by Burlingham and Freud (George Allen & Unwin Ltd.), from *Maternal Care and Mental Health*, by J. Bowlby (World Health Organisation) and from the article "Residential Management as Treatment for Difficult Children: the Evolution of a Wartime Hostels Scheme," by Winnicott and Britton, published in *Human Relations*, Volume I (Tavistock Publications Ltd.). I should also like to thank Dr. Carey-Trefzer for permitting me to make use of a case described by her in her "Study of War-damaged Children," Published in the *Journal of Mental Science*, Volume XCV.

J.W.

CONTENTS

CHAPTER I

Why Psychology?

PSYCHOLOGY has not long been included in the syllabus of the General Nursing Council for England and Wales. Why then is it now considered an essential subject? One part of the answer was, perhaps, given to me by a young nurse at the end of a course in Psychology for nurses I gave at a large London hospital.

"I used to think," she said, "that when patients were irritable and always wanting attention, they were doing it just to annoy me. But I see now, there might have been all sorts of reasons I didn't know anything about."

Psychology in its simplest terms is the science of understanding about people, understanding why they behave as they do in moments of stress or weakness and why you yourself feel as you do in relation to other people and the demands they make upon you. It is, let me repeat, the *science* of behaviour. In other words, it is not just the commonsense of trying to get on well with people, though that comes into it, but the scientific study of what makes up human personality and the effect upon it of particular strains and stresses.

To the ordinary person the business of walking across a room is such a simple, everyday matter that it is not worth considering. But you as a nurse know—and need to know as part of your job—that it in fact depends on a very complicated co-ordination of nerves and muscles and can be affected by anything going wrong with any part of them. Similarly, how we think and how we feel is affected by many psychological factors. Just as it is necessary for a nurse to know much more than the ordinary person about the nerves and muscles which make it possible for us to walk, and what can go wrong with them, so it is necessary for the nurse to know more than the ordinary person about the psychological processes which affect behaviour. This is so because the relation between physical and psychological well-being is so close.

Psychological illness can show itself in what appears to be physical illness and similarly physical illness can and very often does produce psychological ill-health.

During war soldiers can sometimes, as is now well known, become paralysed or blind or deaf without any physical injury but as a result of nervous shock. War, of course, puts people under exceptional strain. But similar examples of the effect of psychological tensions on physical health are frequent in ordinary medical experience. For example, to take one instance from my own recent experience, Jerry, a little six-year old boy, developed a peculiarly awkward gait. He dragged his right leg as he walked and showed every sign of a slight paralysis. Careful physical examination showed, however, that there was in fact no organic basis for this lameness. Instead it became clear after further investigation that he was suffering from serious psychological difficulties which were being manifested through a physical symptom.

As a psychologist I am often asked to examine young children who are very late in beginning to speak. For example, Helen was three years old, yet although at that age a child can normally say some eight or nine hundred words and can combine words into simple sentences, she did not speak at all. There could have been a number of reasons for her failure to speak. It is well known, for example, that a child who is born deaf cannot speak without being specially taught because he cannot hear and so imitate sounds. This was one possible physical reason for Helen's failure to speak. The study of psychology has shown that a child must have reached a certain level of mental development before being able to use words and sentences. Helen's speech failure could therefore have been due to an intellectual reason—to her being below the normal level of mental development for her age.

Helen was examined in hospital and it was found that, she certainly was not deaf. Psychological tests of intelligence showed that, far from her being mentally retarded for her age, she was in fact a highly intelligent little girl. A study of the course of her babyhood and infancy indicated, however, that at a crucial stage she had suffered a bad break in her emotional relation with her mother owing to a long and disturbed separation caused by her mother's illness during which, owing to a combination of circumstances, Helen had to be passed from one person to another to be looked after. This break had been so severe and came at so psychologically critical a time in Helen's development that it seemed possible this in itself might be sufficient to account for her delay in speaking. So in fact it proved and it was this, and not either a physical or a mental defect, that was the cause of her failure to speak. Once this was known it was possible to plan a course of treatment and she now talks quite normally.

Such instances illustrate in an extreme form the interaction of physical and psychological factors. But this close relationship is constantly expressed in infinitely subtle and less dramatic ways, particularly in times of illness.

Later in this book we shall have to consider how and why this is so. But just as it is necessary to understand the foundations of physical health before you can nurse the sick, so it is necessary to understand the mental and emotional—that is the psychological—foundations on which a healthy personality is built before you can understand how to help people in times of emotional stress.

It is for this reason that the first part of the course in psychology now prescribed for nurses covers the study of the development of normal, healthy human behaviour and the pattern of relations on which it depends. Only by having in mind a general picture of the normal course of human development can you know what to expect at various ages and understand what lies behind the characteristic behaviour at any particular phase of development.

The first part of this book, therefore, describes the course of human development characteristic of the majority of people. I have divided the study into the following significant phases:—

(i) Infancy.
(ii) The pre-school child.
(iii) The school child.
(iv) Adolescence.
(v) The young adult.
(vi) The period of middle age.
(vii) The period of old age.

The typical pattern of normal human development has been plotted by psychologists during the study of large numbers of people at every age in the course of psychological research over a great many years. As a result we now know what stage of development is 'normal' for a child at any particular age, not merely by an every day observation of 'ordinary' children but quite scientifically by the detailed analysis of an immense amount of data. But while it is useful for those whose job it is to care for people to know roughly what can normally be expected from them at various stages in their development, it is important to remember that these so-called 'developmental norms' simply tell us what can be expected from the *majority* of people of any particular age.

To take a very simple example. At one year old a child can normally be expected to be able to say clearly two words besides "Mama" and "Dada". At two years he can say about two hundred single words and, even more important, he can combine up to three words into simple sentences. But we must always remember that there is wide variation in the levels of individual achievement. So that although *most* children of two will have reached this stage in the development of speech some will reach it earlier and some later. Small deviations from the norm are not important. A big deviation may, however, as we saw in the case of Helen, be significant of serious trouble and it is part of the purpose of psychological study to be able to recognise when the deviation from the normal is so great as to call for expert advice.

It is also important to remember that while it is useful to divide the study of the development of human behaviour into significant phases we must always remember that there is no hard and fast dividing line between one phase and the next. We cannot, for example, say, "This child is now twelve months old, therefore he has now left behind the phase which we have called 'Infancy' and become a 'Pre-school child'." Each phase of development merges imperceptibly into the next and individuals vary greatly in the rate at which they pass from one phase to the next.

Finally, although it is convenient to refer to "the infant", "the child", "the adult" and so on, we must always remember that there is no such person as '*the* child' or '*the* adult' but only many individual children and adults. It is this recognition that each individual is a unique personality who must be approached and understood and helped for himself alone that lies at the core of good nursing as it does of all human relations.

Frequently when I have been lecturing on subjects such as are discussed in this book, nurses have asked me: "How do psychologists find all this out, and how do they know it is true?"

Psychology is a comparatively young science. But although the knowledge and understanding of human nature on which the study of psychology throws light continues to develop and is continually modified and extended by newer research and study there is already a firm body of knowledge on which there is general agreement among psychologists.

Much psychological knowledge has, as I mentioned earlier, been built up through years of careful observation of the mental growth and personality development of groups of children by teams of trained research workers.

A notable example of this kind of study for instance has been carried out by Dr. Gesell and his co-workers at the Yale Clinic of Child Development in America. Gesell made a very full and detailed study of all aspects of the growth and the development of a vast number of children from birth onwards. He used careful scientific procedures for observing and recording the behaviour of infants and children both in their responses to test situations and in their spontaneous behaviour.

From this careful observation and record Gesell has been able to present in detail the typical stages of development of young children—from birth through childhood.

There have been many other studies of children and the course of their development. In the Institute of Child

Welfare, Berkeley, California, for example, a team of workers has made a detailed study of some 250 young people each one of whom has been tested and observed from birth through childhood and adolescence. Every aspect of their development has been carefully recorded and it is possible to learn a great deal about mental health and development from an examination of the material thus obtained. This is just one example of the kind of research studies carried out, not only in America but in this and other countries also. Studies such as these, carried out with scientific care, make valuable contributions to our understanding of human behaviour.

Just as in medicine much knowledge has been gained regarding physical health and ways of safeguarding it as a result of the treatment of the sick so we have learnt a great deal about what conditions are necessary to ensure that people grow up to be mentally healthy and emotionally stable by studying those children and adults whose development has gone wrong. In such studies attempts are made to go back over the childhood and early experiences of a particular group of people who show in some way that their development has been damaged. An example of this kind of study is that by Dr. John Bowlby of a number of young thieves. In this study Bowlby went into the early history of forty-four delinquents whose delinquency took the form of stealing. He compared the events of their lives with those of a similar group of children, the same age, sex, intelligence level and social economic background. This 'control' group as it is called, were also disturbed children but they did not show their disturbance by stealing. Dr. Bowlby found important differences between the two groups, differences in their basic personality and character and also differences in their experiences during early childhood. He found that many of the thieves were what he described as 'affectionless' characters, lacking in affection or warmth of feeling for anyone. He said of them, "They fail to develop loving ties with other children or with adults and consequently have no friendships worth the name." And further, "There were no roots in their relationships." It is significant that there were none of these 'affectionless' characters in the control group.

He found also that seventeen of the thieves had suffered long separation from their mothers (or the person who substituted for mother) during the first five years of their lives. This also was a significant difference between the two groups.

I have described this study because it is a good example of the kind of contribution to our understanding of behaviour that such careful research studies make.

This is but one example of a great many such studies.

The disruption of family life during the war and the separation of children from their parents through evacuation offered opportunities for research psychologists to study the effects of these experiences on children. For example Dorothy Burlingham and Anna Freud made a careful record and comparison of the growth and development of infants cared for in a residential nursery with that of infants living in their own homes with their own families. This study throws interesting light on the developmental needs of the young child and points to ways in which, where it is inevitable that the child must be brought up without his own parents and home, his essential psychological needs can be provided for.

These are examples of specific research projects designed to throw light on a special aspect of development. Much has also been learnt about the meaning of behaviour by the treatment of psychologically sick people.

Some sixty years ago the great Viennese doctor Sigmund Freud working with sick patients formulated the theory that much in human behaviour results from emotional reactions and conflicts of which the patient himself is not wholly aware. He believed that through experiences in early childhood people developed patterns of behaviour and attitudes which remained with them right through to adult life. He attributed much mental sickness and its consequence in physical sickness to the failure of satisfactory emotional development in early life. He found that by helping people to bring back to consciousness the feelings and memories of their past life it was often possible to help them to gain some insight into difficulties in their relationships as adults. In this way patients were helped to free themselves of much of their unrealised inner conflict and consequently became happier and healthier human beings. This form of treatment by Freud and his followers is called 'Psychoanalysis'. Many others have been stimulated by his work but do not hold his views without some modifications.

It is outside the scope of this book to discuss Psychoanalysis and its ramifications further but I mention it because it has undoubtedly made a very great contribution to our psychological thought regarding human behaviour and human needs. It has enlarged our knowledge because an essential part of psycho-analytic treatment necessitates the revival of memories of feelings and attitudes going far back into early life. In this way the mental and emotional life of the child can be seen through the interpretation of the neurotic or psychologically sick adult. It has therefore stimulated research, deepened our understanding and coloured much of our thinking.

The formation of the pattern of human development

begins with the beginning of human life. Psychologists have long been agreed that the development of a healthy, mature and stable adult depends primarily on the steadiness and warmth of mothering experienced in infancy. That this is so has been emphasised even more strongly by a recent report on researches into the welfare of homeless children made for the World Health Organisation by Dr. John Bowlby.

We will begin our study, therefore, by considering what happens to personality development during the first year of life.

CHAPTER II

Infancy

HOW we behave and what we do at any point in our lives depends not only on what is happening to us at the time but also on all the experiences that have happened to us before. It is these experiences, shaped and fashioned by the inherited qualities we bring to bear upon them—the interaction, in other words, of what we are born and what we experience—that makes us the kind of persons we are. The way in which we deal with things that happen to us depends on the stage of our physical, mental and emotional development.

The story of the development of human behaviour begins with the very beginning of life. It is the story of the human being's growth from the complete dependence of babyhood to the comparative independence of manhood or womanhood and in it the things that happen during the first year of life are of lasting importance.

The period of infancy comes to an end between the twelfth and eighteenth month of life when the infant has developed the main important skills on which every human being's independent existence is based. When the infant has become able to take solid food and has been weaned, when he is able to move by himself from place to place without being lifted and carried by other people, when he is able to make his wants clearly known by the beginnings of speech and to understand the simple talk of grown-ups to him, then the period of infancy has begun to merge into that of the toddler or pre-school child.

In this book we are primarily concerned with the growth of mind and feelings, that is with the psychological development of people and the way they behave in their relations to other people. All through our lives this is closely bound up with our physical health and well-being. Sir Russell Brain, President of the Royal College of Physicians put it clearly in his Rede lecture in 1952: "There can hardly be any bodily state which does not to a greater or less extent influence the mind and there can hardly be any state of mind which does not in turn influence in some degree the functions of the body".

At no stage in human development do we see the physical emotional and intellectual aspects of growth more closely interwoven than during the period of infancy. In this period of beginnings, also, we see most clearly how every human being is part of the world into which he is born. Nobody can grow up in a vacuum and for healthy growth we must have the right kind of human, as well as physical, nurture to satisfy our needs.

At birth the human infant is the most helpless of all newly born creatures. But his development and growth during the first twelve months is extremely rapid and quite spectacular changes take place during that time.

In following the process of growth it is important to remember that the child's development of bodily skills, and of speech, his increasing understanding of things and his gradual building up of relations with people depends partly on the natural maturing of his mind and body and partly on the opportunities for learning and experiencing that are made available to him. The psychological term for this natural maturing is *maturation*. By maturation we mean the process of the growth or natural ripening of mind and body which happens within the child himself.

Until the necessary stage of maturation is reached opportunities and urging from without are of little or no value to the child. To take a very simple example: a child only begins to walk when his body has attained the necessary skill in moving his legs and the balance and co-ordination on which the movements of walking depend. No amount of so-called teaching will make him walk before he is ready—that is before his body has reached the necessary stage of maturation. When his body is ready, however, we can, of course, help him greatly by giving him opportunities and encouragement to try by himself and to experience what it is like to walk.

Thus in walking as well as in every other sphere of development a child can be helped greatly in the process of his growth if we can provide for him the opportunities and experiences suitable to his stage of maturation or inner growth. It is valuable, therefore, for those of us whose job it is to care for children to have what might be called a 'working knowledge' of the natural course of a child's development so that we may know what to expect of him at different ages and thus be better able to give him the help and opportunities he needs. This knowledge will also prevent us from putting too great a strain on a child by urging him to try to achieve more than he is naturally ready for.

In his studies of young children Gesell by making a careful record of the changes that occur in thousands of children in their growth and development through each age level was able to establish what is normal in development at each successive month of life. For example an infant who is developing normally can at one month old lift his head briefly and unsteadily. At three months old he can hold his head erect and steady. These are called *norms of development*. They serve a most useful purpose in providing a 'yard-stick' against which variations in the progress of different children can be measured. But it is important that they should be used with intelligent understanding of the factors that can alter their significance. They need to be related to what we can learn of of the circumstances of the particular child with whom we are concerned.

Many factors such as serious illness, absence of the necessary opportunities or lack of the stimulation of a loving relationship with his mother or mother substitute and of all the encouragement and interest that such a relationship brings can markedly retard development.

As an example of this let me tell you about Jane. Gesell gives the following norms for walking:—at one year a child can walk with only one hand held and at fifteen months he can walk a few steps alone. Up to ten months, Jane was a healthy, normally developing baby and was already making serious attempts to walk. At that age, however, she had a severe attack of whooping cough. This retarded her development and walking was delayed with the result that she was not able to walk even with someone holding her hand until she was seventeen months old. If we had not known about her previous development and her illness we might have taken her lateness in walking as an indication that she would grow up to be a backward child. And we should have made a big mistake in prediction. While, therefore, these developmental norms provide a useful indication of the extent to which a child is retarded or advanced or developing normally for his age total all-round development is so complex and is influenced by so many things that we cannot place too great a prognostic value on developmental norms alone at an early age.

It is important therefore to bear in mind that there are

wide variations in the rate of growth and development of normal children, for no two children are exactly alike. Before we go on to consider the growth of the infant's mind and feelings and the development of his pattern of behaviour I will outline briefly the normal course of development during the period of infancy. The phases of development have been described by Gesell under four main fields of behaviour.

1. *Motor behaviour*

By this we mean the growth and development of the child's control and use of his own body. Both gross bodily control, postural reactions, head balance, sitting, standing, crawling, walking and also finer muscular co-ordination, such as reaching for an object, grasping, picking up objects must be considered.

2. *Adaptive behaviour*

By this we mean the growth of the child's understanding of the things around him. We see it in the way he uses his motor skill to extend his understanding of his surroundings. During the first few months a baby does not relate what he feels with his hands to what he sees. A young baby's first way of exploring and learning more about an object is by putting it to his mouth. Gradually, however, he begins to relate what he can feel to what he can see and he is then able to reach out for things and handle them with more precision. With this development of *perceptual-motor* adjustment and the increasing precision with which the child can co-ordinate hand and eye movements in reaching for and manipulating objects his resourcefulness in meeting and adapting to new problem situations increases also.

4. *Language behaviour*

This includes all visible and audible forms of communication with other people, not only the way in which the child communicates but also his growing understanding of what others say to him.

3. *Personal social behaviour*

By this we mean the child's response to people and the gradual growth of his capacity to adjust to the social culture in which he lives.

Any account of development which is separated in this way is inevitably artificial and unreal. All aspects of growth are most intimately bound together. They are taken separately in this account simply for convenience of description.

Gesell described the newly-born infant up to about four weeks old as "in a twilight zone between sleeping and waking". It takes the baby those first few weeks to become adjusted to his new environment.

Movement during these early weeks consists of:—

(i) Reflex responses such as blinking, sneezing, knee jerking, grasping. These movements are complete at birth or very readily acquired and require no conscious attention. Reflex responses differ from acquired skills. They are automatic responses to a specific stimulus.

(ii) Random unco-ordinated movements of all parts of the body. These movements appear to be spontaneous and without purpose but are probably a response to internal stimuli such as changes of feeling during the digestive process.

(iii) Directed activities which the baby very soon develops. There are negative movements such as turning away from too strong a light or movements expressive of fear at a sudden loud noise. Positive movements in these first weeks are mainly movements towards satisfactions, chiefly related to feeding. A hungry baby very soon begins to nuzzle to find the breast when nursed.

By the time the child is four weeks old we can begin to see fairly definite patterns of behaviour emerging. He can lift his head occasionally and very unsteadily. His sucking movements are by now well established and his eyes are beginning to work together for most of the time. He still makes many spontaneous experimental movements but begins to show more general muscular tone.

He stares for quite long periods at large light expanses such as windows and ceilings and begins to follow large moving objects with his eyes. If a bone ring, for example, is placed in his hand he will hold it and he will show some interest in a rattle or ring that is dangled in front of him.

By this time he is beginning to listen for and notice sounds. Although he still has no means of vocal expression except by crying, it is possible to distinguish different notes in his cries according to whether they are due to hunger, pain or discomfort.

He begins to show some interest in the faces of those who care for him and he is soothed when picked up and held warmly wrapped and firm. He appears to feel real comfort and security from calm and confident handling.

At about three months we see quite spectacular changes in the infant's development. He can now hold his head erect and steady. He can roll over from his back to his side and when he is lying on his stomach he can push himself up by his arms. He can now open his hand and he plays interestedly with his own fingers.

His eyes follow a moving object but he can also now turn his head freely to look at different objects that arouse his interest. He will hold a rattle and look at it and handle it playfully.

He now begins to show real pleasure in making and trying out sounds and he begins to coo and chuckle.

He smiles and coos responsively to people and he shows excitement and pleasure as he recognises preparations for feeding.

At six to seven months, the child can sit for a brief moment without support if he is placed in a suitable position. When he grasps a small object he uses all his fingers working together. He can hold two small bricks, one in each hand, for a short time.

He can reach out for a small object, such as a brick on the table, or take a spoon and bang it on the table in play. If a small object is placed on the table near him, he will look at it with real interest and attention.

By now he begins to recognise a few familiar words and can say some syllables. When he is pleased, as for example at the sight of a familiar person, he shows his pleasure by cooing and crowing noisily.

He is able now to distinguish between strangers and familiar friends. He frowns or smiles in response to expressions of displeasure or pleasure on the faces of the grown-ups who care for him.

At about twelve months the child has learnt to walk with some help—holding one hand—and can lower himself from a standing to a sitting position. He can hold a crayon and make a mark with it on paper and can soon imitate scribbling. He can hold a cup to drink from it. He can put a round block into a round hole in a simple form-board. If you give him a brick wrapped in paper he will undo the paper to find the brick.

He is now able to say two words clearly besides "mama" and "dada" and he can understand and obey simple orders such as "clap your hands". He can also understand and obey when he is told *not* to do things. If he does something that makes people laugh, he will do it over and over again with enjoyment. He will also show real anxiety at the sudden disappearance of a familiar and friendly person.

This is a very condensed summary of the phases of maturation, that is of the developmental norms, during the first year of life. They are based on Gesell's studies. These are not, of course, the only studies of this kind that have been made but there is not space here to go into this subject in more detail. Later I will give some references so that those of you who are interested in following this aspect of psychological study further can read more about it for yourselves.

I want now to consider in more detail the emotional and social development of the infant and to trace the beginning of the pattern of human behaviour. This is closely interwoven with and influenced by the child's total development and growth and it is by relating behaviour to what we know of development in all its aspects that it becomes meaningful for us. Let me give a simple example to illustrate this point. We have seen that after the first month of life the infant begins to look with interest at the faces of those who care for him. Between one and five months he gradually develops better co-ordination of hand and eye and greater control over his posture and head movements and with this development his powers of discrimination between different people also increase. Between the fifth and sixth month the infant becomes able to distinguish between, a familiar and an unfamiliar face. At about this time babies begin to show shyness of strangers. I have often heard a mother say that when her baby was young he would go to anybody and she could not understand why he had suddenly begun to frown and even turn away from strangers.

If we relate his behaviour to what we know of the growth of his capacity to distinguish between different people the change in him becomes understandable.

During the early months of life the infant has no conception of reality separate from himself. Everything that happens is related to the satisfying of his primitive needs for food, and warmth and comfort. From the very beginning he is aware of sensations such as those of hunger, satisfaction, heat, cold, muscle movement, pain and pressure. His most intense feelings at first however are connected with feeding. He shows his first signs of pleasure in the satisfaction of his desire to suck and his first display of anger appears when this desire is thwarted. Dr. Susan Isaacs, who, by her own intensive studies, has contributed greatly to a better understanding of the emotions and feelings of infants, emphasised the overwhelming intensity of the impulses and emotions of infants. The young infant lacks control in his affective life because he has no previous experience and little understanding to draw on to help to stabilise his feelings. Describing the young baby Isaacs said "Knowledge is lacking, understanding has not yet begun, but wants and wishes, fears and angers, love and hate, are there from the beginning."

At first, the healthy infant is awake but little except when he is being fed. These primary feelings and impulses related to the mouth are at the centre of the young infant's mental life. The mouth is not only a means of getting nourishment but also the source of his first knowledge of the world outside himself. Whenever a young baby wishes to explore some new object he puts it to his mouth. He not only eats with his mouth but he thinks and increases his understanding by means of his mouth and he also expresses feelings with his mouth. When feeding proceeds satisfactorily the young infant feels content and happy and secure. An infant who is not entirely content sucks his thumb in an attempt to recapture these feelings of security and comfort.

At first the mother is only regarded as a source of food and it is only very gradually that she becomes for the child a separate person with a life apart from his. The strongest emotions are called out by feeding and gradually the infant's love for food becomes bound up in love for the giver of food.

It is in this early phase of complete helplessness that the infant needs not only to satisfy his hunger but he also needs the emotional satisfactions which come from the physical contact of good nursing and make him feel safe and happy. Breast-feeding is an intimate situation for both the mother and the child and it is on this close and emotionally satisfying relation between the mother and her baby that foundations of stable development are laid. Bottle-feeding must be carried out with the same kind of nursing and physical contact if it is to be made to satisfy these emotional needs for in these early months sensation and emotion are for the baby inseparable.

During all this early period the child's feelings and desires are urgent and compelling. He has no sense of time and no past experience to help him to modify his wishes. He wants something passionately with all his being. If he is thwarted or has to wait he is wholly and passionately angry and when he gets what he wants he is equally wholly content again. It is the mother in this early phase who satisfies him but it is also the mother who sometimes has to thwart him and make him wait. Very gradually as he develops, the intensity of his anger and his love and indeed of all his feelings becomes modified by experience. He is more able to control his impulses because, for example, he is able to remember, although only a little and dimly at first, that although he is hungry and wants to be fed immediately certain sights and sounds tell him that he will not have to wait much longer. He is no longer completely without guidance. Memories of similar things that have happened before help him to temper his feelings. He is slowly building up experiences from which he can learn and so feel less anxious about what is happening in the present. The infant can be greatly helped by a regularity of routine. It is easier for him to adapt his expectations to regular feeding and nursing and so develop a confidence in the continuity of his mother's care and love for him.

One of the critical changes for the infant during the first year of life is the experience of changing from the breast to feeding by spoon and cup. Weaning should not be carried out until the infant has developed so far in mind that his mother has become for him a person whose love is shown in many other ways than just by feeding him. Like every other change in a young child's life it is easiest to accept if it is gradual and if he is given time to get used to it step by step. The child accepts it with least difficulty if he has first enjoyed the normal satisfactions of his impulses during the period of suckling.

The weaning period normally coincides with the time when the infant begins to move from suckling to biting. This desire to bite is associated with the beginnings of teething and it is a further indication of the progressive development of the child. Biting can give the child some of the pleasure and satisfaction that he previously found in sucking. It is also an expression of aggressive instincts normal to this stage of development. The need to bite can best be met by giving the child something hard and suitable for him to practise on.

Next to feeding, the infant's most intense feelings probably centre on eliminating. As bowel and bladder control are not normally achieved until some time towards the end of the second year, we will leave discussion of toilet training to the next chapter.

Quite apart from their importance in physical health and hygiene, feeding, washing, toilet cleanliness—in fact, all the physical care that is given to a young baby—are a part of the love relationship that grows between the baby and his mother. It is on the satisfying quality of this relationship that the foundations of the child's health are laid. We saw that as the baby develops the mother gradually comes to mean to him a separate person on whom he depends for love and care in all sorts of ways and not just as a source of food. At first the baby needs her wholly but towards the sixth month with the growth of his perception he is able to discriminate among people and his affection and interest extends to his father, to his brothers and sisters and to the other people who make up the family circle. He begins to be aware that other people, too, have claims on his mother and by the time he is nine months old he begins to show that he feels jealous of the people with whom he must learn to share her.

During the early months of his life the baby spends most of his life in sleep but gradually he is awake longer and by the middle of the first year he will often lie awake contentedly for quite long periods looking at the things around him or watching his own fingers.

Towards the later part of the year he shows a desire for human companionship. He likes to be with his mother and to watch her as she moves about her work and he has begun to know his place in the family circle as a result of the affection shown for him by his parents and his sisters and brothers. He still, however, depends very closely on his mother and his security and confidence is soon shaken if he is separated from her for too long.

If human babies are to grow up to be mentally healthy adults, capable of good relations with other people, able to accept responsibility and take their proper place in the world they must be given a good start. Psychological research directed towards understanding the development of human behaviour has shown that this 'good start' in life depends first and foremost on the satisfying nature of the bond built up in the early months of infancy between the mother and her baby. Dr. Bowlby describes this bond as arising from "the kind of care which a mother gives without thinking . . . all the cuddling and playing, the intimacies of suckling by which the child learns the comfort of his mother's body, the rituals of washing and dressing by which, through her pride and tenderness towards his little limbs, he learns the value of his own. His mother's love and pleasure in him are his spiritual nourishment".

When this bond had not been satisfactorily formed or has been interrupted through separation there is permanent damage to the personality development of the human being.

In their comparative study of infants reared in a residential nursery with those reared in their own home Burlingham and Freud found that during the first five months of life the babies in the nursery gained weight more regularly, had fewer intestinal disturbances, had clearer skins and a healthier general appearance than the babies reared in their own homes. This they attributed to "more carefully prepared food; plenty of air; less economy in laundry; skilled and regular handling and removal from the disturbances of a proletarian household in restricted quarters". They noted, however, that the breast-fed babies were better off than the bottle-fed wherever they were.

During the second half of the year, however, it was clear that the residential child's loss in emotional satisfaction outweighed the gain in bodily care. The babies in their own families showed greater liveliness and better social response. They were more advanced in reaching out for objects and in active play, they were more active in watching the movements of people in the room and more responsive to their leaving and entering, since whoever came or went was known to them and concerned them in some way. In a residential nursery or a baby ward, on the other hand, there are inevitably many changing personalities and the infant cannot easily come to recognise and differentiate amongst them all.

We saw in our study of the normal development of an infant that between the fifth and sixth month the baby at home develops this ability to distinguish between the changing expressions, the faces and voices of people and this is an important developmental step in the forming of relationships between the infant and his immediate family circle. A child in a residential nursery who does not have this opportunity for the intimate relation with his mother and later with his father and the small and clearly defined family circle is slower in developing this emotional response to individual people. Burlingham and Freud go on to say, "Even where our residential babies are stronger and healthier, these differences in intellectual and emotional development are sufficient to make the private baby appear more 'advanced' and therefore more satisfactory. The comparative backwardness of the residential baby at this stage is due to the comparative unfulfilment of his emotional needs which at this age equal in importance the various needs of the body".

This is but one of very many studies that have been made of infants deprived of a normal home background. I have quoted it in some detail because the importance of its findings cannot be too greatly stressed particularly for nurses of young children in hospital who are inevitably deprived temporarily of the security that stems from the continued presence of their own mothers.

In a later chapter we shall consider ways in which nurses can lessen the damage and sense of loss that this separation can cause.

CHAPTER III

The Pre-School Child

BY the time that the period of infancy is at an end the child who has had a good start will already know and feel happy with, first and foremost, his mother, then also his father and his brothers and sisters. He will be aware of himself and them as separate individual people and he will feel safe in his place in the family circle. He will have begun to learn that he cannot claim his mother's attention exclusively and he will have begun to realise that he cannot always have his immediate desires gratified but must learn to accept some frustration.

By this time also he will have grown away from the complete helplessness of the newly born baby towards becoming an active vigorous little child who can move about his world a little unaided. He will be able to crawl and walk with help towards things that are out of his reach and to pull and reach out to handle things that interest him. He will recognise familiar sounds and faces and he will be beginning to understand what is said to him simply. He will be taking solid food and drinking from a cup and will be starting to try to express himself in words.

The second year of childhood is in many ways a period of consolidating the skills which the infant has learnt during this first year of rapid growth. This 'toddler' year is, as it were, a bridge between infancy and early childhood proper. Although the child is beginning to move towards greater independence he is still very dependent on his mother and the good feeling towards him that is shown not only by her but also by the others who make up his family circle.

He still needs to have his mother near him for most of the time when he is awake and to feel sure of a steady and dependable background of affection. It is only from the security of this background that he can safely move towards greater independence and in this way extend his knowledge and understanding of the world around him.

Let us now look briefly at the course of his development during this second year.

Around 15 months he can stand alone and walk a few steps without help. He begins to be able to use a spoon. He can place one brick on the top of another. He can say four or five words clearly and he uses also a great deal of expressive 'baby-talk' or jargon. He shows interest in and tries to help when being dressed.

By about 18 months the child is much surer in walking and does not have many tumbles. He can climb on to a chair and seat himself. He can put a number of small bricks into a cup or box and can hold four or more of them at a time. He can turn the pages, two or three at a time, of a fairly thick-paged picture book and he is beginning to look with interest at the pictures and can usually point to the picture of one familiar object when asked, e.g., "Which is the dog? Show me the dog."

He finds great pleasure in scribbling with a crayon. He is now able to feed himself, though somewhat messily, with a spoon. By now he can say about six real words, but he still chatters a great deal in his own jargon.

He co-operates eagerly in being dressed and undressed and loves to try to do things for himself.

At 21 months or so he can walk backwards as well as forwards. This marks a very important advance in his development of muscular control and balance. He is beginning to be able to make a circular movement with his crayon as well as the straight strokes of his earlier scribbling. He now joins two words and sometimes three into sentences and loves repeating short sentences that are said to him.

He is beginning to distinguish shapes more clearly and can fit not only the round piece but also the square piece into their proper holes on a simple formboard.

By this age bowel control is usually established and the child will ask for toilet attention.

At about 24 months the child can run, can walk up and down easy stairs without help and can build a steadily-standing tower of six bricks. He begins to be interested in practising finer manipulative skills such as, for example, cutting with scissors. He can turn the pages of his picture book one by one. When shown a picture card on which are five common objects, namely, a dog, shoe, cup, house and clock, he can name three out of the five of them and point to each of the five when asked.

He has many more words, about 200, in his vocabulary and he uses three-word sentences to describe his own experiences—"Bobby fall down"—"Pussy take ball". He is now beginning to love listening to stories, nursery rhymes and jingles and looking at pictures and being told simple stories about them. In his play with his doll or teddy bear he begins to imitate the events that he knows about and experiences in his own life. He plays at feeding his doll or teddy bear and putting it to bed and he mimics the grown-ups he knows in his world.

By now, at any rate during the day, bladder control is fairly well established and he often remains dry at night also.

He asks for food, drink or the toilet.

This very brief outline gives some idea of the skills and achievements that can be expected of a normally developing child during the second year of life.

We can perhaps best understand something of the emotional needs of the child during this toddler year of one to two, if we refer again to the comparative study made by Burlingham and Freud of infants without families and of those brought up in their own working-class homes by their own parents. In this comparative study it was found that the institution child in the first two years was at a disadvantage wherever the emotional tie to the mother or to his family is "the mainspring of development". They found that toilet training and the development of speech during the second year of life are closely related to the child's emotions and that successful achievement in these spheres depends largely on the satisfactory quality of his emotional relations with his mother (or mother substitute) and his immediate family.

Let us consider first the way in which training for toilet cleanliness comes about. The development of bowel and bladder control marks a significant step in social adaptation. It is important to recognise, however, that it is not easy for an infant to learn to retain his urine and faeces and it is a serious mistake for those who have children in their care to treat the excretory functions as though they are mechanical or reflex processes that are quite separated from the child's emotions. The question of the best time to begin toilet training is one over which there has been and still is much controversy. Many people hold the view that training in establishing clean habits cannot be begun too early. Only this week I visited a mother of a three weeks' old baby who told me that she already had what she called "a battle of wills" with her baby every day over using the pot. This young mother was convinced that if she was firm enough and persistent enough she would triumph over her baby and that before very long the "miserable business" as she described it of washing soiled nappies would be at an end. Experience has shown, however, that if toilet training is begun too early and too strictly there is frequently a breakdown in cleanliness at a later stage in development. Habit training cannot be treated as if bowel and bladder functioning were merely reflex actions. As with every other aspect of behaviour psychological factors enter into this also.

As we saw in the chapter on Infancy, in the first few months of life a baby's chief pleasures are pleasures of the senses and among these are the pleasurable feelings experienced in sucking and eliminating. We saw also that at first a baby cannot distinguish between his love for food and the comfort it brings and his love for the giver of the food. Therefore the process of weaning from the breast or bottle cannot be begun satisfactorily until the infant has developed to the stage where he is able to recognise his mother as a separate person whose love for him is shown in many other ways as well as by the giving of food. When he has developed far enough to realise and feel this he can accept the changes involved in weaning without undue distress. Similarly toilet training can only be carried out successfully when the child's emotional development has progressed to the stage when he is able to set store by and appreciate the satisfactions to be gained from trying to do the things that give pleasure to his mother or the person whose good feeling for him he values most. Toilet training, like every other aspect of early training in social adaptation, is closely linked with a child's feelings for the person who undertakes the training. He is ready for this training, then, when he is old enough to *want* to co-operate with his mother in developing clean habits, when his mother's good feeling towards him, her smile of pleasure at his successful control, means more to him than the instinctual gratifications which he needs to control in order to win her approval of him.

The achievement of bowel and bladder control therefore grows out of the gradually developing understanding by the mother of her infant's needs. The young mother who was determined to train her child to be clean during the first few weeks of life was really riding roughshod over the baby's own development in these matters. She was too impatient to give herself time to discover her baby's natural rhythm and in this way she was interfering not only with the beginnings of a natural process for her child but also with that loving and understanding relationship between the mother and her baby which is the foundation on which healthy development is built.

As with every other aspect of development children vary widely in the rate at which they achieve toilet cleanliness. They vary in the readiness with which they can understand the adult's suggestions of time and place. Whenever training in cleanliness is achieved during the early months of life it is based on reflex action—the child's *muscles* are responding mechanically to a stimulus but his mind and his feelings are too immature for him to be ready to co-operate with his whole being. Such toilet cleanliness is at the best precariously maintained and at the worst can be truly damaging to his mental health by putting the child under the too great strain of having to accept adult standards long before, in his total development, he is ready for it.

It is best achieved when the mother can match her expectations for control to what the child's level of growth makes him capable of. The child should be able to feel that he has the steady support and help of his mother as he tries to develop control. Like most acquired adaptations it is slow and difficult of achievement and it remains for some long time bound up, as it were, within the circle of the mother-child relation.

It is some long time before bladder and bowel control is divorced from this feeling relationship and becomes purely automatic. During early childhood a breakdown in toilet cleanliness is an indication of a break in the child's relation with his mother or the person who acts as the mother substitute. One of the problems of billeting that was met with during the evacuation of children in the last war arose from this kind of breakdown in toilet cleanliness. Even many school children who were experiencing separation from their parents for the first time wet their beds and soiled although they had been completely clean at home for many years. It was as if this control could only be maintained through the support that living close to their parents gave them. To most of these children this breakdown in control was deeply distressing.

For the pre-school child control is, because the achievement of toilet cleanliness belongs to an early phase in his social and emotional life, liable easily to lapse again when something happens to disturb him in his emotions and to disrupt in his feelings the bond between himself and his mother. This often happens when a child is overwhelmed with jealousy at the arrival of a new baby in the home. Describing the reactions of Margaret aged 2½ years to the new baby her mother said "When she first saw me nursing the baby she just stood there and made a puddle on the floor! She hadn't done that for months before."

Let us turn back now to the toddlers without families in the residential nursery to see how they fare. Toilet training with these children was found to be prolonged and difficult if the child was cared for by many different nurses or if he disliked the nurses who handled him. Children whose training for cleanliness proved specially difficult could finally achieve cleanliness only if they were taken over for a time by one person. It was also noticeable that children could maintain their good habits of toilet cleanliness when in contact with certain nurses but broke down again completely when helped by others.

This all goes to emphasise the importance of the personal relationship of the young child with his mother and the support that it gives him during this early period when he is building up inner control. If we realise this it should be easier to understand and therefore tolerate the child whose separation from home and parents causes lapses of this kind when in hospital.

Failure to achieve toilet cleanliness or a breakdown in toilet habits when under emotional stress are common symptoms of psychological ill-health. From treating these cases in the psychological departments of hospitals we learn how closely this aspect of human functioning is bound up with feelings and emotions. We have seen that a young child's breakdown in cleanliness is often an indication that he is probably feeling himself thrust out to an independence from his parents for which he is not yet ready. It is sometimes an expression of aggressive feelings—a weapon for attacking his parents when he is angry or bears a grudge against them. Like other symptoms of dis-ease it is not a conscious or deliberate action but something that arises from very primitive emotions and over which the patient has no conscious control.

We shall refer to this later when we come to consider problems related to human behaviour in illness, because the complexities of human behaviour shown by adult patients in hospital have their roots in patterns of development formed in very early childhood.

Speech during the second year is the other area of development in which the institutional child fares worse than the child who is brought up in his own home. This retardation in speech development is not noticeable during the first year when the infant finds so much pleasure in trying out sounds for their own sake.

It was found by Burlingham and Freud, however, that though their babies in the nursery showed an average rate of development in speech in the first year, during the second year their speech development became progressively slower so that by the age of two even those children who were well up to average or even forward in other ways were some six months retarded in speech.

There would appear to be two reasons for this. Speech is learnt partly by imitation and the young child at home is the only non-speaking member of his family where speech is the main mode of communication with other people. The young child in his own home, therefore, has much more opportunity to learn to speak by imitating his brothers and sisters than has the toddler in a nursery, who is for much of his time surrounded by other toddlers who also cannot speak.

There is, however, another factor which is probably much more important. The real incentive to speak is in order to have a means of expressing oneself and communicating with the people whom one loves in the world outside oneself. It is part of the emotional interplay between the child and his parents.

During this toddler year a young child in his own

family usually spends most of his day playing near his mother who talks to him as she works, and it is out of this close contact of the young child with his parents that the urge to imitate and use speech grows. So closely is speech development during the second year related to contact and good relationship with the mother that children who suffer separation from their mothers quite frequently lose this newly acquired ability to speak. That was what had happened with Helen, the little girl whom I described in Chapter 1. When I first saw Helen, she was three years old and she did not speak at all. Her baby brother was born when she was two, and for the next six months Helen had been separated from her mother who had spent most of the time in hospital. It seemed, when she was two, that Helen was going to be a real chatter-box. When her baby brother was born Helen stayed happily with her Grandmother of whom she was very fond. But when the mother became ill Granny could not look after both Helen and the new baby while their mother was away, so Helen was pushed around from one person to another during the next six months. By the time her mother was well enough to be home again with her children Helen was not speaking at all. This complete regression shows how deeply Helen had felt the rejection, as it seemed to her, by her mother and her granny at a time when there was no other adult in her world because her father was in the army overseas. It also emphasises the young child's need for a continuing close relationship with his mother and immediate family circle.

During the second year the young child spends most of his time in activity for its own sake. This is the period when the child is trying himself out, exercising his newly found capacity to move freely and to gain mastery of balance in standing, walking, running, climbing and jumping and thus to develop greater motor control. In this sphere of development the toddlers in the residential nursery were found to have an advantage over those in their own homes where space for movement was much more restricted and there were more things that might damage the child and also more objects which the child had to be prevented from damaging.

Here is a description of these children in the nursery. "At this period for a while they disregard all toys and show little interest in their companions; they behave as if they were drunk with the idea of space and even of speed, they crawl, walk, march and run and revert from one method of locomotion to the other with the greatest pleasure. These children mostly use toys where they can include them in the continual game of movement. Sometimes for an hour on end the whole population of the Junior Toddler room is on the move, circling round, crossing and recrossing like people on a skating rink. Handling, of course, is not confined to toys. Whatever is loose in the room (whether coal bucket, nappy bins, broom, pail, etc.) is included in the interest and is handled and explored. If permitted, the children use to the full the newly-developed functions of opening, undoing, pulling out and especially unscrewing."

Children who have the freedom to develop their control of hands and legs in this way not only experience great pleasure and satisfaction in their growing skill but also quickly become able to do things for themselves and to move towards greater independence. As their muscular control increases so their confidence and self-reliance grows with it. This need for activity and freedom to explore and experiment is characteristic of the whole of the pre-school period. We do these young children a great dis-service if we deny them opportunities to develop in this way. We all know those adults who insist on holding the child's hand and try to make him walk sedately when he wants to try to run and jump. In attempting to guard the child from tumbles and hurts, they are violating his natural urge to grow.

Throughout the whole of the pre-school period children show unending zest in practising and perfecting their bodily skills. Whenever the healthy young child is awake he is naturally active, always 'on the move' and never still for more than a few minutes at a time. By the time he is five, therefore, he has gained considerable mastery in his muscular skills and his movements are balanced and controlled.

This is also the period in which rapid development of fine muscular control takes place. At three years the child has moved from mere scribbling to being able to copy a circle and at three and a half he can copy a cross. By this time he can not only fit large shapes into their appropriate places on a formboard but also small pegs—round pegs into round holes and square pegs into square holes. By the time he is four he has developed sufficiently fine muscular control to be able to copy a square which is a much more difficult task than drawing a circle. If you ask a three-year old child to draw a man, he will probably make a large circle, two strokes for legs and two rounds inside the circle for eyes. By the time he is five he will be able to draw a man with head, eyes, body, arms, some suggestion of hands or fingers, and legs.

The young child gets real satisfaction from doing things, drawing, painting, cutting with scissors, threading beads, trying to put on his own shoes, dressing himself and doing up his buttons.

We can help children at this age by providing for them suitable material for play and opportunities to do things which will increase their skills. It is of major importance that those who job it is to care for young children should have some knowledge and understanding of the course of their development so that they can know what kind of tasks are suitable. The other day I saw an old sampler done in incredibly fine stitching into which was sewn the name SALLY, AGE 5, 1794. As the date on Sally's sampler shows it was done a long time ago. In those days it was thought to be good training for a young child to learn to sit still and do very fine sewing. But we know now that to make a young child sit still and struggle with tasks that make quite unnecessary demands on the undeveloped co-ordination of hand and eye is to violate grossly the ways of a young child's growth.

In providing young children with suitable occupation, therefore, we should remember the general trend of maturation. The larger movements ripen first and the finer skills much later. A baby of eight months will use his whole hand with all his fingers working together to grasp a small object but by the time he is a year old he will show much more precision of movement and will be able to use just his thumb and finger to pick up a pellet.

We must, therefore, not make a young child feel tired and frustrated by giving him things to do which run counter to this natural order of development. If the occupation is to thread beads give the young child big, coarse beads and a thick lace on which to thread them and leave the fine needle and thread and the small, delicate beads till he is older. Similarly if he wants to draw give him a thick crayon that is easy to grasp and a large sheet of paper on which he can draw with those big sweeping movements which are of the kind suited to his developmental level and let the refinements of movement and grasp come later.

This pre-school period is not only an age when the child enjoys activity and movement for the development of muscular control but it is also a time when his sense perception is rapidly developing. This shows itself in his curiosity about everything around him. He is interested in forms and shapes and colours, in sounds and texture and sizes. His knowledge of space and distance grows by seeing and touching as well as by the experiences gained through the child's own movements. Just as in the development of motor skills control over larger movements come first, so at first the child can only perceive large differences in size and distance; more refined perceptions come later.

Children from two to five find great satisfaction in play material that affords opportunity for the development of sense perception. At this age they think and learn and reason, in short their intelligence and their experience grows and develops, through doing things, through manipulation and very largely by touch. It is only by handling real objects, fitting nests of boxes one inside the other, playing with sand and water, pouring water from one vessel to another, filling, emptying and refilling tins with small objects, that the child builds up his knowledge of the world around him. At this time the sense of touch plays quite as important a part as sight and hearing. A young child learns much more by handling things than by being told about things or looking at them. Children who are allowed freedom to handle things in this way very quickly become skilful in doing a great many things for themselves. That is why it is unfair to a child to prevent him from opportunities of learning by his fingers. To keep saying to a child, "Don't touch" is indeed bad advice, for just as in infancy a baby uses his mouth to learn and explore and in that way extends his understanding and experience, so the young child learns and thinks with his fingers, through the 'feel' of things. It is only later, when he has gathered knowledge and experience of real things that he can begin to be able to think in words.

Similarly a young child first learns about numbers by counting real things. It is only by counting and handling real things that abstract numbers begin to have some meaning for him.

During this period of development and particularly between two and three years old, the use of language develops rapidly. When the desire to communicate with people has been aroused by a good relation with his parents the speed with which a normal child develops his speech after about two years of age depends not only on his intelligence, though that is of major importance, but also on the opportunities that are available to him for exercising and extending his skill. Children of 2½ to 3 years take a positive delight in naming things and repeating short phrases. At this age they begin to relate phrases to actual situations and enjoy the constant repetition of a phrase that has meaning for them. Mary, aged 2½ was standing on her mother's knee while being dried after her bath. As she stood, looking over her mother's head, her mother remarked, "Look, Mary you're bigger than Mummy". Mary seized on the phrase with excitement and after that for some weeks she said it each evening, adding to its range. First she said, "Bigger than Mummy, bigger than Daddy". Gradually she extended it to include all her toys and pets. "Bigger than Teddy, bigger than Pussy" . . . and so on bubbling over with delight as she thought of each new phrase.

Although as the child grows from three to five his language and his ability to make his wishes and his thoughts and his ideas known by words is continually increasing his talk is for the most part an addition to thinking by doing, rather than, as with grown-ups, a tool of thought itself. The child's ability to reason in words develops slowly as his ability to use language grows. The young child can only deal with problems that can be solved by actual handling of the concrete material immediately available. He can only work out that two and two make four if he can count up the four objects that are there to hand. After three years a reasonably intelligent child begins to think in words and can therefore begin gradually to draw on the experience of other people and deal with problems not actually present for him to see and handle. This is the time when the child, so eager to know and understand asks so many questions. "Why?" "What's that?" "What is it for?"

It is a mistake, however, to think that because a young child can speak so well his thought processes are the same as those of an adult or that words necessarily convey to the child the meaning that they have for us. All through the war years while Margaret's daddy was fighting abroad, her mother tried hard to keep alive the thought of 'daddy' in the child's mind. Every day she used to lift her up to look at the photograph on the wall and point to it and say, "There's Margaret's daddy". When Margaret's daddy really came home again, Margaret looked at him in dismay and said, "You're not my Daddy. My Daddy's on the wall."

Janet aged 4 had been in hospital for a week. She had fretted badly and was looking forward eagerly to being taken home. During that week a new car her father had ordered had been delivered and he proudly drove it to the hospital for her when the time came to take her home. When he arrived Janet, who was all expectant, overheard a nurse say, "Janet's father has come for her but it's a pity he's taking her in an open car." And when he came to get her, Janet, who had been longing for this moment, burst into tears and refused to go with him. Finally when all coaxing failed he carried her to the car screaming and resisting. When she saw the car and was wrapped up warm and comfortable in it she soon became happy again. Nobody could understand the meaning of the outburst until many years after when Janet was grown up and explained it herself. She said that she had never seen an open car before and she thought that it would have no sides at all and that she would be bound to fall out and be lost. This had happened at a time when being in hospital had aroused in her feelings of rejection and anger against her parents for leaving her there. Her fears were increased because she had often been bitterly jealous of her father and wished to be rid of him so that in her confused feelings it seemed that he too must wish to be rid of her also.

These are just two examples of the kind of misunderstanding of meaning that words can convey to a young child who has no background of experience on which to draw. It happens very frequently.

That is why we should make the answers and explanations we give to a young child in hospital as simple and concrete as possible.

We have seen that this period of one to five years is a time in which there is very rapid growth in every sphere of development, in physical skills, use of language, powers of perception. It is not surprising, therefore, to find that at the same time very great advances in social and emotional development also take place. In many ways this is a most tumultuous and difficult period for the young child. In her account of "The Psychological

Aspects of Child Development" Dr. Isaacs has said, "In the period of from one to five years in particular, emotional difficulties occur so frequently that they may be looked upon as normal to this phase of early childhood. Few, if any, children do not manifest some sort of difficulty, although these vary very much in degree and in persistence." This is particularly true of the child in the years from one to three. In these early years he has not yet developed the power to control nor the capacity to understand his feelings which are often very intense and overwhelming. During this period of early childhood he has a very limited experience of reality on which to draw for reassurance and comfort. And until he gains more knowledge and understanding of the world of reality around him he has nothing to draw on to help him to temper and modulate his feelings.

By the time he is able to move from place to place and is beginning to talk, he will have come to know both his father and mother as *persons*. He will have begun to recognise that they are not always there, ready and waiting to satisfy his immediate needs but that they are people on whom other claims as well as his are made. As his interest in things and other people increases he is gradually able to loosen his hold on his mother though he cannot bear too long a separation from her. Too long a separation arouses in him a frightening sense of isolation and he has not yet enough experience to feel sure that people and things that he cannot see do in fact still exist. His feeling of isolation when his mother is out of sight or hearing for too long a time can be very terrifying to him when he is still small.

As the child moves towards greater independence the ways in which he comes into conflict with the wishes of his parents inevitably increase. When parents, as they must, thwart and frustrate the child's instinctive desires this arouses anger and hatred in the child. In the young child these angry feelings are very complete and overwhelming while they last. These feelings of hatred can be very terrifying because of the intensity of the sense of guilt and shame which they create even in a very young child.

Perhaps the most difficult problem of adjustment for the young child arises from difficulties in adapting himself to his place in the family. During babyhood the bond between the child and his mother is very close and she quite rightly places first his claims on her care. Gradually, as he grows from babyhood, he has to yield to the claims on her made by the other members of the family. Jealousy is a very basic emotion and the problem of dealing with the feelings of rivalry for his mother's affection arouses a great deal of anxiety in the small child. Because he loves his mother he wants to have her all to himself. When she gives her attention to other people he is quickly overwhelmed by feelings of anger and hatred towards her. This feeling of hatred towards someone whom he loves and on whom he is so dependent is a very terrifying feeling, particularly as young children cannot be quite sure how much real damage these angry feelings can actually do and are therefore afraid of the power of their own wishes.

Very early in life children begin to feel conflict between love for their mother and love for their father. A great many fears of young children arise from their jealousy of their parents. All children pass through phases in which they are more deeply attached to one parent and jealous of the other who seems to them a rival for the affection of the one whom for the moment they want all to themselves.

We have seen that during infancy and early childhood, the child's most important relationship is with his mother. During this time the father provides the economic and emotional support necessary to enable the mother to care for her baby in an atmosphere free from worry and disharmony. Gradually, as the child grows older, both parents are known and loved by him as separate persons but the proverb "Two's company, three's none" applies to the feelings of young children as well as of adults and there will be many times when he wants his mother or father all to himself and cannot bear to share. Because the child's love for his parents and his dependence on them is very great, jealousy of them is one of the most upsetting experiences. But it is part of the growing-up process of every child.

As the child grows he may have to recognise the position of brothers and sisters in the family and accept the very real claims made on the parents by the other children. Perhaps the most difficult change for a young child to accept is that brought about by the birth of a new baby into the family. Here the child is faced clearly with a second rival for the mother's attention and love. And however carefully and wisely the child is prepared for this event it is not possible entirely to prevent jealousy being aroused and with it the hatreds that inevitably follow from it.

This finds its outlet in many different ways. It is best for the child's mental health if his parents can maintain an understanding and tolerant attitude to these outbursts of anger when they come, so that the child can feel unconsciously that they are helping him through this difficult time when his bad feelings get the better of him and that the warmth and constancy of their feeling for him remain unchanged. In time then he will learn to share the affection and interest of the parents with the other members of his family and accept his own position in the family.

If, however, his jealousy and hostility are driven underground by punishments and fear of losing his parents' love they will find expression in anxieties, night terrors, fear of the dark or in regression to more infantile habits such as thumb sucking, a breakdown in toilet habits, or the making of countless demands on his mother.

Buried jealousies and hatreds in childhood often show themselves in adult life in resentments and discontents which bring about failure to make and maintain good human relationships. Conflicts and tensions during these years of early development are natural and inevitable. In the security of a loving and dependable home background the normally developing child works through them and resolves them and it is on these affectionate relations of early childhood that the pattern of behaviour in adult life, in love and marriage, family life, work and friendships, is laid.

As the young child grows up and his interests and knowledge and experience extends he becomes progressively less at the mercy of his immediate impulses and feelings. He learns to consider more than his desire of the moment and to recognise the claims of other people. One of our most important needs throughout life is to have friendly relationships with other people and very soon a child begins to recognise the reward in friendship of observing and trying to adjust his own wishes to the things that please and displease the people whom he loves and who make up his world.

By the time he reaches school age he should, if his early development has been satisfactory, feel secure in his home relationships and, from the safety of this feeling, be able to show friendliness towards adults and other children. He should be eager to learn and be reaching towards new experiences. He should be able to meet some disappointments and frustration without being overwhelmed by them.

The five-year old child is still very vulnerable. His control over his body and his feelings is easily upset. He has as yet very little background of knowledge against which to judge a new and difficult experience. In his life in a grown-up world he is inevitably constantly reminded of his own littleness and inadequacy. And there will be many times when his primitive feelings of hatred and anger will overpower him in spite of the support that his parents give him. There will still be times when he will lose confidence in his parents, however good they are in reality, and in himself as a person worth loving.

We have seen how young children are helped in periods of stress most of all by the security that is fostered by their parents' patient understanding and dependable ways with them.

All children have also within themselves a valuable guardian of their own all-round development. This is their capacity for play.

Adults whose job it is to care for children, whether healthy or sick, need to understand and appreciate the great importance of play in a child's development.

Before considering the development of the school child, therefore, we will discuss the use and value of play in the normal development of young children.

CHAPTER IV

Play in Childhood

FOR the young child play is not merely a means of relaxation. It is the main business of his life. Froebel, who devoted his life to the study of the education of young children, spoke of play as not merely a means of passing time, nor mere activity, but as the means by which "the child's innermost nature must be satisfied".

It is through play that the young child develops his bodily skills and increases his knowledge and understanding of the world around him. Through play his thinking becomes clearer and more constructive and he is also helped in his progress towards a more controlled state of feeling. By playing with other children the child learns to give and take, to develop interest in and friendliness towards other children. In his play with other children he meets real problems of social adjustment and he learns independence in meeting them.

Those whose job it is to care for children need to understand the importance of play in their development and be able to make suitable provision for it.

The nurse of sick children in hospital can use play as a powerful ally in helping a child to settle down happily and to make steady progress towards recovery from his illness.

Let us consider first the play needs of the normally healthy child. Opportunities for play for the physically sick child in hospital are not, of course, the same but need modification and adaptation and these we will discuss later.

In order to understand the play needs of children at differing ages we must relate them to what we know of their progressive development and growth.

In considering the course of development of the child throughout infancy and early childhood we saw that good care of the child at any stage of growth involves regard for every aspect of his development—the growth of his bodily and muscular skills, his sense perception, his speech, his thinking, his feelings and his friendliness towards other people. Every aspect of the child's total growth is served by differing forms of play. In her comprehensive study of "Play in Childhood" Dr. Margaret Lowenfeld observes, "There is play that expresses the bodily impulses of the child; that apperceives his environment; that prepares the child for life; that enables him to mix harmoniously with his fellows."

We have already seen that a child develops best if he is encouraged to make use of his maturing abilities at what we have called the natural maturation phase of the child's growth. The way in which a child plays also depends on the needs of his development at any particular period. We can help him best by providing the right opportunities for play and play material suitable to each phase of his development.

The earliest kind of play takes the form of bodily activity. As early as at two months a baby begins to play. He finds delight in kicking in his bath and whenever he is awake he lies in his pram waving his arms and making spontaneous, undirected movements. Later he plays with his own fingers and toes and it is by this kind of play that he learns to realise and use his own body. He watches the movements of his hands and feet as he lies and he gets pleasure from watching the movement of other things also such as the trees and the changing shadows made by the movement of clouds. Although much of his watching is passive it is usually accompanied by a great deal of spontaneous bodily activity.

We have seen also how the young child learns to speak by first of all playing at making sounds. By the time he is three months old he begins to show positive pleasure in playing at making new sounds and in noticing the effect of his 'speech' on the people around him. At six months he coos and crows to express his pleasure.

It is through his play that the infant begins to learn about his world. He discovers what things look like, what things feel like and how people react to the different noises he makes and the different things he does. And all the time he is learning more and more about the feel of his own body and steadily acquiring greater motor skill.

Later he shows a playful interest in people; he loves to be talked to and sung to and begins to show need for companionship in play. From about nine months he loves to take part in repetitive games such as Peep-bo and Pat-a-cake. From such games as Peep-bo he has the satisfying experience that even when a familiar and loved face is hidden from view the person has not left him completely but can reappear at a moment's notice. It would seem from every infant's delight in this game that he gets some symbolic satisfaction from playing it over and over again and finding every time that someone who appears to be lost can be rediscovered.

From four or five months the infant is able to enjoy a few very simple toys such as a rattle, a string of brightly coloured beads, a rubber toy for his bath, a bell, a spoon, a cuddly toy. Later he will find satisfaction in toys which require judgment and manipulation such as hollow boxes or bricks that fit one inside the other, or rings of graded sizes to be fixed on to a round peg. Any toy given to a baby should be suitable for sucking but not so small that he could swallow it.

Towards the end of the first year and also throughout the pre-school years a child needs toys that will help him to develop his maturing senses of touch and sight and hearing so that he can use them to learn from first-hand experience about distance, size, shape and sound. This is what he is doing when he balances bricks one on top of the other, bangs with his spoon on his tray, picks things up and drops them again, crowing with delight at the noise they make.

Not only does such play develop a child's muscular skill and sense perception but, because of the pleasure and satisfaction in his own achievement it brings, it also helps to give him emotional stability and assists his progress towards greater independence.

Throughout the whole of the pre-school period the urge to develop his motor skill and sensory perception very largely determines the kind of play that the child finds most absorbing.

We saw that until the child can really master the skills involved in walking and running and climbing and balancing much of his time is taken up with moving for its own sake. But gradually he includes in this moving around some manipulative tasks, pushing and pulling carts and horses and prams, or even practising the extra skill in balancing demanded by carrying some object in each hand as he walks.

When Jane, aged 20 months, was given a small doll's pram she spent a whole hour solemnly pushing it quite empty backwards and forwards the whole length of the nursery, skilfully turning it to avoid any furniture or object that came in her way, her face rapt with pleasure.

The elderly lady who had given this present to Jane was disappointed that she did not, as she said, "use it properly". She wanted her to tuck up a doll in the pram before she started her 'walk'. And she could not understand that Jane was using the toy to meet her need of the moment, to extend her skill in walking and balancing and judging distances and space as she guided the pram to avoid bumping into other objects.

Children of two still have much to learn about spaces and distances and the relative sizes of different objects. They are fascinated by problems of manipulation and love fitting variously shaped blocks into their appropriate holes, putting little stones into a tin or packing bricks into a box, tipping them out and doing the whole thing over and over again. Pouring water from one vessel to another is an absorbing job to children of this age and it is only by playing in this way that they begin to be able to judge when a vessel is full. A little girl of two when given a mug of milk used to take it up and pour it slowly all over the tray watching with complete absorption while the milk trickled through the cracks of the tray and ran down on to the floor.

Her mother thought this a clear demonstration of the child's wilfulness and naughtiness but, watching the child's rapt attention as she poured, it was clear that here was a problem that she simply had to explore. Of course it was most inconvenient that she should have chosen to find out about liquids and pouring with the good milk that she should have been drinking but it was easy to satisfy her interest by letting her play with water in a large zinc tray with numerous tins of varying sizes so that she could pour water from one tin to another until she was able to judge when a tin was full and to stop pouring if she did not want it to overflow.

Very soon the same little girl could fill up her own mug with milk from the jug without spilling at all.

Throughout the pre-school years play with water and sand provides un-ending pleasure to the child.

As the child develops, his skill in finer manipulation also grows and he begins to find pleasure in painting, drawing, threading beads and doing similar tasks which require a greater mastery of hand and eye co-ordination. All the time, however, increasing skill in larger movements is being achieved through play.

Play material for the pre-school child, therefore, should be the raw materials for experimentation, materials which the child can learn to master and in so doing extend his experience and understanding of the world around him. The child needs opportunities for play with water, sand and earth; plasticine, paints and crayons, bricks, wooden pegs and hammer and other simple tools —simple sense training materials from the use of which he can extend his knowledge of sizes, shapes, colours, distance and sound. The young child is full of curiosity and lively interest in many things. Play which stimulates his interest and his efforts to find out about things which arouse his curiosity help forward his thinking, for as we have seen previously a young child thinks largely by doing things with his hands.

This kind of play, therefore, not only increases the child's manipulative skill but also fosters his power of understanding and the development of his thought.

All constructive and manipulative play gives the child pleasure and satisfaction in achievement and this in turn increases his confidence in his own abilities. As his understanding of the things around him is increased his world becomes for him a more dependable and less frightening place.

Imaginative play or 'make-believe' also figures largely in the play of the young child. The imaginative play of young children is always interwoven with phantasy. The young child, whose language ability is not yet far enough developed to enable him to express his thoughts and feelings adequately in words uses play as a medium of expression and a means of sorting out his thoughts and experiences and inner wishes. These are among the most important ways by which a child's harmonious emotional as well as social development is served by imaginative and phantasy play.

For young children, imaginative play serves as a bridge, as it were, leading from manipulative thinking to the more adult way of thinking by means of language.

Even as grown-ups we know how much we are helped by thinking over many of the things that happen in our lives. Experiences that have seemed bewildering and difficult when we were living through them become more understandable when we have had time to 'live through them' again in our thoughts. How much more necessary is it, therefore, for the young child to be able to go over in his own mind some of the bewildering problems and experiences that he has to meet. He does this by playing out his experiences again imaginatively. Most children re-create in make-believe play those experiences that have seemed too bewildering and difficult for them to grasp all at once while they were happening. In their re-creation of them they will frequently express their feelings about them, feelings that are often quite different from the reality of the situation.

For some weeks after Mary started school, she used to 'play out' the whole school day's events when she came home. She seemed to have to do this before she could settle happily to any other play. And watching her as a person who knew the school well it was clear that the whole scene was distorted by Mary's own feelings about it.

Mothers have often told me how their children who have been in hospital, play at 'hospitals' over and over again on their return home and how in their play they present the nurses or doctors as severe and punishing persons when in reality they have been mild and gentle. But what the child is really expressing is how threatening and alarming the whole experience seemed to him and how angry and aggressive were his own inner feelings.

Children use imaginative play to reconstruct not only unpleasant and difficult experiences but also pleasurable, happy ones. By living over happenings again in play they give themselves time to sort them out and lessen the intensity of the first emotion that the real experience aroused, make themselves master of it and so absorb it into their total experience. Over and over again they play out the family situation, being mummy or daddy or the new baby—sorting out in varying ways the events of their own lives.

Just as a child learns about the *things* in his world and at the same time develops new skills by manipulative play, so in his make-believe and phantasy play he gains in insight and understanding of his social world at the same time as he advances towards more control and mastery of his own feelings by means of his play experiences.

The young child is little and dependent in a big world. Always to be the little one, the one who needs helping or the one for whom all the others have to wait because he cannot do things so quickly, is often frustrating and irritating. In make-believe play the young child finds a temporary escape from the pressures of his environment. For a while he forgets that he is little and becomes an important, big person with a real job to do—a policeman, a soldier, a mummy or a daddy, a nurse or a teacher. In this way he gives himself an escape for a brief time from his own inferiority and weakness and gains in personality development in the process.

Make-believe play, however, serves for the child an even more important function than this. We have seen in our study of the development of the pre-school child that he experiences considerable emotional stress during these early years.

By make-believe or imaginative play a child is able to give expression to, or, to use a psychological term, *externalise* some of his inner feelings. For the small child who has not yet much experience of reality against which to test and modify his inner emotions play provides a safety-valve—a means whereby he can maintain inner harmony and balance. When a child plays at being a daddy or a mummy or a big and powerful person who has gone out to shoot giants or tigers he is not only helping himself to learn about and solve problems of the social relationships and behaviour of grown-ups, he is also giving expression to, and in that way finding release for, some of the pressure of emotion within himself.

During these years of growing-up a child inevitably meets with frustration and thwarting which fill him with resentment and angry feelings towards the person who is caring for him and whom he loves. There are times in every young child's life when, though normally loving and friendly, he hates his parents and wishes they would die—although afterwards he will feel bad about it and wish he could make amends. These are very frightening feelings for a young child to have. He does not really know yet whether thoughts like that can make what he temporarily wished actually happen. To find himself wishing to be rid of the person whom he most needs and depends on in all the world is terrifying. It is also confusing and disturbing to find himself mixed up between loving and hating the same person.

Here again imaginative play provides the child with a way of expressing some of his feelings and inner phantasies in a safe way and so helps him to grow towards a more harmonious state of feeling. Without his consciously realising what it all means play of this kind has a symbolic meaning which provides an outlet for pent-up feelings.

Instead of getting mixed up between hating and loving his real mother he can get rid of the bad mother of his feelings in his make-believe play of pushing the nasty old witch into the oven. Instead of hating and wishing to attack and kill his big and powerful father, whom he also loves, admires and needs, he can play at being Jack and kill the giant. In this way he can put outside himself, or externalise, the bad feelings within him and get rid of them in a way that prevents him from harbouring feelings of guilt which can be destructive to the developing personality.

The intensity of this sort of feeling and its reality for a young child was demonstrated very clearly in the course of a clinical study of war-damaged children who attended the Child Guidance Clinic at the Hospital for Sick Children, Great Ormond Street, London. The study was carried out by Dr. Carey-Trefzer and is reported in full in Volume XCV of the Journal of Mental Science. One of the puzzling things about the children whose records were followed during the course of this study was the fact that some children who suffered very real and terrifying war-time experiences quickly regained their emotional poise and showed no permanent damage to their stability while others showed extreme and persisting reactions to events which were, as far as could be judged, not in any way sufficiently devastating to explain the permanence of their effect on the children.

One little girl, Sheila, at the age of five had been in a hospital with whooping cough when the hospital was hit by a bomb. She was not injured at all physically. And although some of the other children were injured none were killed.

On returning home Sheila was entirely changed in her behaviour. She was withdrawn and showed no feeling for or interest in her family and home circle. For two weeks after the bombing incident she completely ceased to talk. Even after that she talked very little and frequently refused to eat.

When she was eight years old she was referred to the local Child Guidance Clinic because she was making no progress in school and was very shut-in. She was excessively quiet and showed very little expression of emotion. Her failure in school work was in no way caused by limited intelligence for her intelligence on testing was found to be very much above the average for an eight-year old child. Sheila lived in a fairly well-knit community in a suburb of outer London and the hospital was a small one which had served that area. Of all the children who had experienced that bombing incident, Sheila was the only one who had been referred to the Child Guidance Clinic on account of nervous troubles. It was difficult to find out why Sheila had been so severely upset by an experience which had not caused such persisting upset for any of the other children.

Sheila had never talked at all of the bombing incident so that her mother could not give any more details of what had actually happened. Before that time Sheila had apparently been developing normally and presented few problems. When she was five a baby brother was born. Sheila showed no jealousy and her behaviour had not changed. A few months later, however, both children developed whooping cough and as the baby was very ill indeed it was then that Sheila was sent to hospital to be nursed while the baby was nursed at home. She had not seemed to mind this arrangement at all.

Treatment at the Child Guidance Clinic began when Sheila was eight. During the first two months of regular weeky attendance very little change in her behaviour was observed.

After two months, however, a casual question while Sheila was playing prompted her to tell of the hospital incident: "I could never forget it—I thought they were all killed—the nurses carried us out—I was the first one out—there were great heaps of glass everywhere—I was terribly upset—I was the first one out—I was the first one out!" Although Sheila was then asked other questions about the incident she answered each by shouting, "I was the first one out."

From this time Sheila's mother began to see some improvement in her at home. Her play at the clinic now became very aggressive and noisy and she played a game of 'bombs' for some of the time each week.

It was only after eight months of treatment at the clinic that she was able to talk freely about the hospital incident. She described the whole incident again and said, for the first time, that it was because she had had to go away while her mother kept the baby at home that she had felt so "awful". By now she was able to discuss her feelings quite freely and she said frankly that she had felt she hated Mummy and the baby and wished they would die. She went on to tell that she felt like that about everybody when she was taken away to hospital.

When she was asked what she thought when the bomb fell, she almost shouted, "I thought it *had* happened". Indeed she thought her wish had come true.

It was during the few minutes after she had been taken to safety and was there alone, "the first one out" that she felt sure that all the other children had been killed and she alone was left. This was exactly what she had wished and it was terrifying.

The terror of experiencing, as she thought, how powerful her own wishes could be produced the kind of reaction which was to be expected. She ceased to talk, she refused to eat, she showed no active feeling at all. She was attempting, in fact, to withdraw from a world where to have wishes and feelings could prove so dangerous.

I have quoted this case in some detail because it illustrates how acute can be not only a young child's hatred but also his dread and his guilt.

We see in this case study how greatly Sheila was helped in her progress towards recovery by play, how week after week she had to live through this whole experience again and again in her game of 'bombs'.

It is important, too, because it shows so clearly how the normal pattern of Sheila's behaviour was distorted by the chance coinciding of hidden psychological conflict with a terrifying real experience. If we had not been able to find out about her inner conflict, we should have wrongly thought that she was a child who was much more vulnerable in the face of physical danger than most normal children in wartime proved to be. In fact if this bombing experience had happened to Sheila some months earlier, before her baby brother's birth, it is probable that she would have gone through it undamaged, like the other children in the hospital. Equally if she had not had the frightening real experience of the bombing which made her feel that her 'bad' wishes had such potency she would probably have been able to resolve her own inner conflict and find release for her feelings of jealousy by means of imaginative play in her own home, because basically she was a mentally and emotionally healthy little girl.

Children up to the age of two years do not show much active interest in joining with other children in their play. Even when a group of toddlers are playing in each other's company, they do not often play *together* in the way in which older children delight to do. But although he plays his own game a toddler also watches and imitates what other children do and gradually begins to take part for a little while in their play. By the time he is five he can play quite happily as one of a small group. It is this companionship with other children in play that supports the young child in working out his feelings and inner phantasies together with other children free from the interference and domination of adults. By playing with other children and experiencing the give and take which that involves he learns social adaptation in real situations at a level which he can understand. It is by real experience of active, social play that the child gradually learns to modify his inner feelings and phantasy as he relates them to the real world that lies around him and that increasingly claims his interest.

It can be truly said, therefore, that adequate opportunities for play during childhood are a vital necessity to the growing child if his total development is to be satisfactory.

Although, for reasons that are obvious, many kinds of play and some toy materials, also, are quite unsuitable for the sick child in hospital, with some adaptation and thought, many opportunities for play can be made available to the child who is not too ill for any effort of this kind. Interesting studies have been published of the suitability and uses of various kinds of toys for hospitalised children in the pediatric wards of some American hospitals but provision for play in hospital must depend on the ward routine of the particular hospital concerned.

Because play is so important a function of childhood, I will end this chapter with one or two general observations that can be applied by any nurse in any children's ward.

To be of practical use in hospital toys must be easy to clean and sterilise and to store. They must neither be noisy nor require strenuous physical exertion. In offering toys to children the nurse should bear in mind the developmental level of the child and where possible the child should be allowed to do his own choosing.

Although many children get satisfaction from toys which give them something to do and which challenge their manipulative skill and provide occupation we must not be disappointed or put out if the child uses a toy in a totally different way from that intended. Toys seem to have special meanings to different children and they use them according to their need.

Because children in hospital are undergoing a specially traumatic experience they will particularly welcome toys that provide scope for phantasy play: families of dolls, nurse and doctor sets, tea-sets and all kinds of domestic articles, miniature trains, cars, aeroplanes, farm and wild animals, a few bricks, odds and ends that can be used in various ways. Children will use these toys in the ways that seem most important to them to act out some of the pressing events in their own lives and by giving expression to some of their own fears and loneliness as well as their angers and hatreds find relief from feelings that press too heavily on them.

Imaginative play is very real and vivid to the young child; so real indeed that phantasy and reality often become confused in a child's mind and it is difficult for him to distinguish between the two.

Just to illustrate how real phantasy can be, let me tell you about Peter and Sally. Sally was 3 and Peter 4 and they had been playing happily and quietly together for some time when Sally rushed to her mother imploring her to come quickly because the tigers were going to eat Peter all up and they could not send them away. Sally's mother went with her immediately to the nursery and found Peter crouching in a corner with a look of real terror on his face. He was only reassured when she had entered into the whole make-believe drama and helped to drive the imaginary tigers away.

Jack, another little boy of my acquaintance, had to go away to hospital when he was 3½. He had taken with him his old baby shawl which he always cuddled in moments of stress—by this time a very bedraggled and tattered piece of shawl indeed—but for him "Shawly" was very much more than a shawl. Fortunately, the ward sister with real understanding appreciated the importance of Shawly in Jack's world and made friends with it as well as Jackie. She allowed Jackie to have Shawly with him all the time. One night, after a very disturbing day for Jackie the nurse on duty heard peculiar noises coming from Jackie's bed, "Pop, pop, bang, bang." Jackie was sitting up in bed sucking his thumb for comfort while with his other hand he held the bedraggled old shawl up and explained to nurse that Shawly was shooting all the giants.

In both cases it would have been easy to ridicule those

children and say that they were just being silly because there were neither giants nor tigers there. But because phantasy is so mixed up with reality for little children and the fears were very real to them they could only really be helped by taking the giants and the tigers seriously, by letting Shawly and Sally's mother, for example, drive them away while at the same time recognising that the tigers and the giants were an expression of real fears and stresses which the children needed help and support in combating.

Finally because their play is so real and so absorbing to children we should try if possible not to interrupt it or break in on it too suddenly. This is not always easy under the stress of hospital routine. But the nurse can usually find ways of giving the child some warning that the time for packing up the toys is approaching and so help him to prepare himself for bringing his play to an end.

CHAPTER V

The School Child

STARTING school is a big event for every child. Let us stop for a moment to consider what the five-year-old child is like and how well equipped he is to meet this new adventure.

By the time the child is five, providing all has gone well for him and his early development has been normal, he will be a sturdy little person, active and full of energy. He will have increased considerably in his muscular skills and his sense perception though neither the development of his senses nor the control and co-ordination of his muscles will be in any way complete. The acuity of a child's vision, for example, continues to improve up to about the age of eleven and, what has been described as "muscle sense" which is the awareness of one's own movements by means of sense organs in muscles, joints and tendons, continues to develop in sensitivity up to about the age of thirteen years.

It is not surprising, therefore, that throughout early school life children need abundant opportunities for movement and activity.

Activity for the five-year old is not confined to bodily movement, he is busy and active also in his thoughts. His thinking is constantly being stimulated by the things he is doing and investigating for himself. By the time he is five, he can talk clearly and he asks a great many questions for by now his speech is becoming a positive help to his thinking.

In his feelings he is growing away from the tempestuous lack of control that is so characteristic of the years of early childhood and he has become much more stable and less easily disturbed. Even when he is upset in his feelings it is much more easy for him to overcome his conflict and regain his emotional poise. He is steadily gaining in the capacity to tolerate frustrations and to deal with difficulties more independently.

If he has been happy and secure in his relations with his own parents and brothers and sisters he is now able and ready to extend his interest and feelings of friendliness to people outside the little world of his own home. Although he likes the company of other children and enjoys playing near them he is still very dependent on adults and, at any rate during his early days at school, he tends to transfer his dependence from his parents to his teacher. Her approval or disapproval of what he does matters much more to him at first than the friendliness or unfriendliness of other children. The healthy five-year old, then, is ready and eager to meet the new adventures that beckon him but, although he is now not ill-equipped within himself for this venture, his real security is still anchored in his home.

The developmental period which we are now considering ranges roughly from 5 years, that is the beginning of school life, to 12 years which marks the onset of puberty.

This covers the whole of the infant and junior school period. Although, as I have stressed previously, we must never fall into the error of thinking that any period of human life can be sharply divided from another it is perhaps convenient to consider the two periods separately. The development of children from roughly 5 to 7 years, which for English children is normally the time spent in the Infant School, is marked off by fairly distinctive characteristics from the later years of 7 to 12, the time usually spent in the Junior School when for most children more formal schooling begins.

Perhaps the differences between the two periods becomes clearer if we regard the early period as one of transition or as a bridge between the pre-school period and the characteristic period of the school child proper.

As we should expect children during their time in the Infant School are not so confident nor so stable in their feelings as are the older school children. We have to remember also that, except for children who have been in nursery schools, they are at this time experiencing the first big break with the sheltered environment of home. For many children this can arouse considerable anxiety. Separation from their own mothers, the overawing quality of a strange and often a large building, meeting for the first time larger groups of children to whom they are often strangers, all that is involved in attaching themselves to a different adult whose ways they do not really know—all these make big demands on children's capacities for adjustment. It is quite common to find children developing mild anxiety symptoms such as sickness, headaches, disturbed sleep and frightening dreams or fretfulness and excessive dependence when starting school.

The ease with which a child meets and accepts this new and big experience depends on the steadiness of his earlier emotional development and the extent to which his basic security is firmly established.

Although after five the emotional life of the child steadily becomes more stable and less intense the growth away from the tempestuousness and difficulty that we saw was so characteristic of the pre-school years takes place slowly. The emotional difficulties and turbulence which found expression in the second and third years in temper tantrums give place to obstinacy and defiance.

Although children in the Infant School are still very dependent on grown-ups it is a dependence that steadily diminishes as the child becomes progressively more capable of sustained co-operation with other children.

The five-year old child is still very much wrapped up in himself. His world is centred in his own feelings. His own needs and wishes are far too urgent for him to be able to see things from the point of view of other children. If you watch a young child playing with other children you will see that he is often much more absorbed in his own phantasy than in the wishes or ideas of the other children. Although children of this age like to have others playing near them and it may seem from a cursory glance that they are playing in groups on closer observation it is clear that each child's play within the group is very individualistic. Small children will play contentedly with others so long as this play suits their own purposes and the other children fit in with their wishes. They do not really play *with* children in any co-operative sense but use other children as they might use toys as pawns in their own individual game.

Mary, a little five-year old girl expressed this very clearly, though perhaps unwittingly, when she had been staying away from home with her Aunt for what seemed to her a long time. She had missed her own toys and the little girl, Maisie, who lived next door. When the end of her holiday came and she was at last really going home, she rushed up and down the room chanting with delight: "Home to Maisie and all the other toys." And that really expressed what the other children meant to Mary aged five—a part of her own play material.

Gradually, however, children begin to play *with* others

in the sense that they begin to be able to see things from other children's points of view and modify their own wishes accordingly. By the time the child is seven he is able to co-operate with other children in play in the real sense of co-operation and he becomes more and more capable of playing with a group of children for quite a long time without needing the presence of an adult for support.

This movement away from the dependence on adults for love and protection marks a very important stage in the child's growth towards the complete independence of maturity.

The Infant school child is still very much given over to imaginative and make-believe play and, as we saw in our study of the play of the pre-school child, the five-year old's imaginative play has often very little relation to his real experience. It is rather an expression of his own inner feelings and quite different from reality.

Very gradually, however, during the Infant School period children begin to devote less and less time to phantasy play. Imaginative and make-believe play becomes more related to reality and takes on the form of dramatising or acting. As the child's own real experiences increase he is more able to relate new experiences to real happenings he has known about in the past. As he becomes less dependent on his immediate family for emotional satisfactions and his relationships are spread over many people, especially his own contemporaries, the intensity of his primitive feelings is lessened and he is more able to organise and control his feelings. As his grasp of reality and experience of real happenings extends he is gradually able to develop a truer sense of proportion and with it more tolerance for the mistakes and faults of others.

The young child, up to about six years old, is often much harder and less tolerant in his judgments of other children than grown-ups would ever be. Just as in their phantasy play they often, as we saw, show as make-believe parents a harshness and severity quite unrelated to the kind of treatment they have themselves experienced in their real lives, so also they cannot temper their judgments or keep them in proportion. Whether they are praising or blaming another child they carry their praise and their blame to excess. Dr. Isaacs suggests that by being so harsh in their judgments and setting such severe standards they are really supporting themselves against their own clumsiness and lack of skill. It is as if the young child cannot dare to be tolerant of weaknesses in other children until he is more sure of his own control. So we find him pointing with scorn to the child who is sobbing in terror and saying, "Isn't he a cry-baby?" or to the child who is really distressed because he has accidentally soiled his pants, saying "Dirty boy. What a dirty boy he is!"

Young children whose skills are not yet securely established are not always able to prevent themselves from wetting or soiling when under the stress of great emotion, they are not always able to keep from crying when they are frightened or unhappy, they cannot always restrain an outburst of temper when their anger gets the better of them. And by being severely critical of another child's lack of control they are really criticising their own weakness.

This pattern of behaviour persists in many adults, who tend to be most critical of other people for the very faults which they themselves possess. Even while criticising they get a certain satisfaction and support from finding the same weakness in others.

As the child's play relationships with other children widen and his experience of real situations increases so he is able to bring a truer sense of proportion to modify his judgments as well as his feelings. He is beginning to learn what it is like to play and work with other children and he learns when to make demands and when to tolerate frustrations, how to give and how to take in his relation with his own contemporaries. He begins to find in other children allies, and, with the support that this comradeship brings, he is able to move away from dependence on adults and the dominance of adult judgments and values.

Although this change takes place slowly throughout the Infant School years the seven-year old child who is ready to move on to his Junior School is a very different person from the five-year old just entering school. Not only does he find in his comradeship with other children support against the domination of the influence of grown-ups but he also finds in his play with other children satisfactions and interests in the real world which give him some release from that inner world of phantasy which often weighs so over-poweringly on the younger child.

By the time he is seven or eight the child enters a period which, if his earlier development has been satisfactory and all has gone well, is likely to be the most stable time of his childhood—a pause before the ferment of adolescence begins.

Let us now consider what are the main characteristics of the school child during these middle years of seven or eight to twelve.

Already in our study of the changes that take place in the personality and behaviour of the younger child we have seen that these changes are bound up with and always influenced by the child's total all-round growth and development. Similarly the characteristic needs and pattern of behaviour that emerge during these middle years of childhood can best be understood if we bear in mind that they arise out of the interweaving of the emotional, mental, and physical aspects of growth.

By now the child's world is steadily widening and more people and interests are entering into it. This lessens the intensity and the conflict of his feelings towards his parents. He is also physically much less dependent on them because he can do so much more for himself. Consequently that close emotional relation with his parents which was necessarily so great a part of his early childhood has gradually been reduced.

Out of his wider experience he is now able to tolerate disappointment and accept some frustration. And because of this he is able to have sustained relationships with other children. Perhaps one of the most striking characteristics of the school-child from seven years onwards is his decreasing dependence on grown-ups. He gradually shows that he neither needs nor desires to share his experiences with adults but rather turns away and becomes more and more reserved in his relations with them. He regards them with a more objective judgment and is able to be quite critical of them. In order to wean themselves more completely from dependence on grown-ups children support themselves in their break by forming gangs and secret societies which adults are excluded from sharing.

Strengthened by his comradeship with other children and the real social relations which he is experiencing the child is able to repress his own phantasy and turn away from make believe to find his satisfactions in real achievements. He is now concerned with the acquirement of real skills and with the pursuit of real knowledge about things and people in the world of reality. This is the age when a child so often asks, when you tell him a story, "Is it a *true* story?" "Did it *really* happen?" "Was there *really* a boy who did that?" And the story gains in value if it is 'really true'.

In his progress through the Infant to the Junior School, the child gradually begins to welcome opportunities for more formal school learning. He begins to want to learn to read and work with numbers and he welcomes tasks that call for positive effort from him.

His eager pursuit of knowledge of the real world leads to considerable increase in manipulative skills and in the use and understanding of language. One characteristic that is common to the whole period of childhood is the love of and need for active movement. Normal healthy school children if allowed to grow freely are almost untiring in their physical activity. Not only do they run and jump and climb and skip, tear about on scooters or bicycles and play ball games but they use their active bodies to find out about things, to learn, to make and construct. And all the time when they are free to do so they shout and sing and talk unceasingly.

I can think of many schools where even yet the children are denied every opportunity for natural activity but one in particular comes into my mind, a Junior School in an overcrowded area in North London. There the children sat still at their desks throughout the whole long morning. They were only allowed to speak when permitted, after putting up their hands. When at last the time for 'break' came, they assembled into lines and marched out quietly without talking. As they crossed what was for them the magic threshold that divided school from the world outside they burst into the freedom and space and began to chatter and run and jump with all the reinforcement of pent-up energy that had been allowed no outlet. I stood with the headmaster and watched them go and he shook his head sadly saying it was a pity that they were so unruly and noisy outside *in spite of the fact* that they were taught such orderly behaviour in his school!

This constant urge towards movement, towards doing things with every part of himself—feet, eyes, hands and tongue—is a child's natural means of spontaneous growth. This need for activity is understandable when we remind ourselves that neither the development of a child's sense perceptions nor his powers of muscular control or co-ordination is in any way complete. It is only through exercising their bodies and extending their experiences in many directions that children can attain the full development of their skills and sensitivity and increase their understanding of the world they live in. The child has a tremendous urge to understand his world and his desire for activity is bound up with his desire to understand. The more he understands his world, the safer and the more independent he feels. And the best way for him to learn is through his own activities, his own social experiences of playing and working with other children; in short, through his own contact with reality.

As the child grows older he prefers to work and play in a group. He loves team games in which he begins to experience the satisfaction to be gained from identifying himself with the spirit of his team and subjugating his own personal desires to the good of the team. Eleven years is the peak age for playing with the 'gang'. The child now begins to show active hostility rather than mere indifference to grown-ups and the authority they represent. And disturbance in emotional development often finds its expression in anti-social behaviour in which some form of rebellion against authority finds its expression.

Children of this age enjoy belonging to groups and clubs—Scouts, Guides, Brownies, Cubs and such like. They love collecting things and enjoy a good deal of communal 'swopping'. This is an age also where there is considerable rivalry and competition, between individuals as well as between gangs and groups, and between boys and girls.

During this period boys and girls begin to separate and go their separate ways, following their divergent interests often with expressions of considerable scorn for the members of the other sex. It is quite usual for boys who, a year or two previously, joined happily in play with girls to begin to pour scorn on the idea that they should ever mix. David aged nine was home after his first term at prep. school. Previously he had joined unquestioningly in play with his sister and her friends but now he preferred to mess about on his own rather than to play with girls.

"Really," he said, when it was suggested that he should join in their game, "you can't expect me to play with hags." Although it seemed that his feelings and attitude were dictated in part by the code of his new school the code itself had developed as an expression of the general trend towards separate interests and the rivalry between boys and girls which characterises this period of childhood.

During later years of childhood there is a noticeable tendency for children to begin to form closer and less transient friendships among themselves and quite outside their own family circle. These friendships mark a new stage in the child's growth towards emotional maturity and they form a necessary part of his emotional development.

If we compare the pre-school child with the child in the middle years of his childhood it can be clearly seen that the part that the adult who is caring for him needs to play is a constantly changing one. The school child is mainly a practical person interested in real and concrete things. Even in hospital where, inevitably, they will be temporarily deprived of normal activities the children's questing interest in the reality that surrounds them can be fed by sensible answers to their questions and reasonable explanation given at a level of simplicity which they can grasp.

Although the school child is mainly concerned with concrete things his interest in ideas and, with that, his growth towards more mature ways of thought develops from his interest in actual things. As he grows towards adolescence he begins to turn from the more practical pursuits of his childhood years and their concern with concrete things towards an interest in ideas and principles and the beginnings of the more abstract thinking of the adolescent.

The child is best equipped for the changes and adjustments required of him in adolescence who has had opportunity to live through his childhood years richly and actively in every way.

CHAPTER VI

The Nature of Intelligence

IN the earlier chapters of this book we have followed the progressive growth and maturing of skills during a normal child's development. We saw, for example, that by the time a baby is six months old he begins to be able to sit up without support and that a child of three years will have developed his fine motor control and co-ordination between eye and hand to the extent that he is able to copy the drawing of a circle. As we have followed the course of the normal development of children we have seen how closely the growth of the child's body and bodily skills is bound up with the growth of his understanding and his feelings. So interwoven are these aspects of development, particularly in the early years, that when we try to judge the quality of a young child's mental ability we base our judgments largely on the total pattern of behaviour that the child presents. We notice carefully what a child can *do*, what skills he has acquired, because, as we have already seen, thought processes in young children largely find expression through physical activity and skills but we also notice how well he talks, how easily he understands what we say to him, how easily he makes himself understood and what his social behaviour is like.

In doing this we are assuming correctly that human behaviour is strongly influenced by intelligence: that is by the capacity to understand and thereby to make use of experience. Because we have the intelligence to understand and learn from experience we can modify our feelings and judgments and, consequently, our behaviour in the light of our new experience and understanding.

Psychologists have for many years past been concerned with studying the ways of mental growth and finding methods of assessing the intelligence or mental capacity of different individuals. One of the striking facts that has come out of these studies is how widely individual people differ in their mental ability.

Now I have stressed previously that a child's sense of security and, as a consequence, his emotional stability increases as his knowledge and understanding of the world around him grows. This is true not only of young children but of grown-ups also. It is an important fact to bear in mind when our job is concerned with people—particularly so for a nurse caring for people who are faced in hospital with new and for them often alarming experiences.

The quickness and ease with which a person can understand and apply what he has learnt previously to his way of meeting a new experience such as illness and being in hospital is dictated largely, though not of course wholly, by his inborn intellectual ability. It is this inborn ability which sets a limit of possibility beyond which each individual's capacity to learn and understand cannot go. This limit varies greatly among different people. Because the development of intelligence is not, however, something that takes place quite separately, in a vacuum as it were, from the individual's total development, a person whose inherent intellectual ability is high does not always reap the full fruits of his original endowment. Recent studies have gone to show how closely the satisfactory development of intelligence depends on both emotional and physical satisfactions during the growing period.

Because intelligence effects behaviour so potently it is important that nurses should not only be aware of the very wide range of differences in the intellectual capacity of different people but that they should also have some understanding of the way in which a person's total development is affected by his inborn mental capacity and of how this inborn capacity influences his behaviour and his ability to cope with the stresses that he meets in life. It is perhaps easiest to understand this if we relate it again to the growing child. Its importance is demonstrated by the fact that when a child is admitted to the department of psychological medicine of any hospital because he has shown by some symptom or another that he is emotionally maladjusted one part of the diagnostic investigation is given over to the assessment of the child's intelligence with as great a degree of accuracy as possible. Measuring a child's level of mental development is a very complicated procedure because intelligence shows itself in so many different ways and is affected by so many differing influences. It is, however, possible for a trained psychologist to make this assessment and to measure whether the child's mental ability is average or in what direction and to what extent it differs from the norm.

The tool of this kind of measurement is called an Intelligence Test.

When we give a person an intelligence test what is it that we are seeking to measure?

The word 'Intelligence' is here used in a rather precise sense. By it we mean a person's capacity to learn and to profit by experience; it is the ability to use what you have already learnt and apply it to the new problems, tasks and judgments which you are called upon to make. We draw on our intelligence for every task we have to do and for every judgment we have to make, whether it is something very simple or something involved and complicated. It has been defined by Professor Sir Cyril Burt as "general inborn mental power". It is described as "general" because it enters into every aspect of behaviour, every kind of task that we do. Although this capacity to learn, this "mental power", steadily develops and matures throughout our period of growth, the extent to which it will develop and mature is determined from birth—that is, it is inherent, or inborn.

The rate at which a child's mental ability grows and develops can be affected by many things: certain kinds of accidents and illnesses, poor nurture, lack of suitable opportunities on which the mind can feed and—and this last is very important—the lack of satisfaction of emotional needs particularly in early childhood. But even if everything possible is done for children and they are given not only the right kind of physical nurture but also opportunities for satisfying emotional relationships and for the extension of social activities suited to their level of maturation we cannot increase this potential maximum which is hereditary and inborn.

It is this inherited potential which we seek to assess by means of intelligence tests. We cannot measure this directly in the way that we can measure a child's height or weight but only by his skills, by what he has learnt or by what he can do. Nevertheless an intelligence test is designed to offset as far as possible the effects of learning and opportunity and to measure not what the individual has already learnt but rather his capacity to learn. The ways by which this is achieved are too technical to fall within the scope of this book. But it is useful for the nurse, particularly of children, to have some understanding of what meaning the results of an intelligence test convey.

The score of an intelligence test is usually expressed in terms of Mental Age. If a boy aged 10 years was given an intelligence test and his score on that test gave him a mental age of 10 years we should know that he was able to do successfully in the test what about 75 per cent of a large random group of children of the same age could manage to do. That is, we should know that his mental ability was average for a ten-year old. If however a boy of 10 years has a mental age of 12 years on the intelligence test that means he is brighter or more intelligent than the average ten-year old and that his achievement in the test corresponds to that of an average child of twelve. Similarly a boy of 10 years with a mental age of 8 years would be less intelligent than the average and able to achieve in the test only what an average child two years younger than himself can do.

In order to make possible comparisons of people of different ages the mental age score is expressed as a "mental ratio" or "intelligence quotient". This is based on the relationship between the chronological or birthday age and the mental age of the person tested. The intelligence quotient or I.Q., therefore, is the Mental Age divided by Chronological Age multiplied by 100.

For our brighter than average boy, whose Mental Age was 12 years this would be:

$$\frac{\text{M.A.}=12}{\text{C.A.}=10} \times 100 = \text{I.Q. } 120$$

The boy whose M.A. was the same as his true age would have an I.Q. of 100 and the dull boy whose mental age was eight would have an I.Q. of 80.

The I.Qs. of most people fall roughly between 90 and 110—that is round about the average. The number of people whose I.Q. deviates widely from the average becomes progressively smaller the further away from the average one gets: both the genius and the idiot are comparatively rare. Because by far the largest proportion of people are around average in intelligence the standards and the demands made by the world are suited to people of average intelligence. People who are very much below or very much above average in intelligence have difficulties and often show problems of behaviour arising from this difference from the normal capacity to understand and fit in with the demands of the world around them.

For example, there are many gifted children whose ways of thinking and reasoning, as well as their speed of learning and understanding, are equal to that of the average for much older children. Unless the quality of their intellectual ability is recognised and responded to they may become irritable and tiresome because they feel so constantly frustrated.

Let me tell you about Michael. He is 9½ and exceptionally intelligent. His I.Q. is 179. His Mental Age—that is his capacity to understand and reason is as mature as that of an average boy of 17 years old. I have followed Michael's school career for some years now. He has never been an easy child. He found it difficult to play for long with other children without becoming impatient with their slowness to understand and would then lose control of himself and wreck the game. He was referred first to a psychological clinic of a hospital by his school teachers because they could not manage him at all. He would not work and no other child would play with him. His parents who came with him to the clinic looked strained and anxious. His mother particularly looked worn out and defeated in the effort of trying to control Michael.

His school mistress said that he was a naughty little boy who would never attend to his work at school so, as a punishment, she put him down into the group below his real age group. The result, of course, had been disastrous. Not only did he continue to pay no attention to school lessons but he employed his able and fertile mind in plotting new ways of making himself a bigger nuisance to his teacher and a torment to the other children. It was at first difficult for his teachers to realise that much of his troublesome behaviour arose from the frustrations he felt when his urgent desire to know and understand was obstructed and remained unsatisfied. When they altered their approach to ways of teaching Michael and gave him much more scope and opportunity to satisfy his questing mind they found that much of his inattention in classwork had arisen out of real boredom and that the only peaceful way to live with Michael was to harness his mental energy to the pursuit of occupations and tasks in which he could recognise some real purpose and which therefore seemed to him worth while.

The last time I saw him he had been in hospital for six weeks and had just returned home. He talked a great deal about his experiences there. Quite clearly one of the things he had found hardest of all to bear was, as he angrily put it, "the way the nurses talked to me as if I was a kid of six".

I learnt from Michael's mother that he had been a great nuisance while in hospital. When in a lecture to nurses I used the case of Michael as an example of the kind of behaviour that can arise when a child is much more intelligent than his own age group one of the nurses said, "Surely a nurse is much too busy to be expected to look up every child's Intelligence Quotient before she starts to talk to them at all". Of course that is obviously true.

But if we can carry in our minds some idea of the wide variations in intelligence and powers of understanding that can be found among children of the same age we can more readily treat each child as an individual person and be sensitive enough to be able to learn from the child's own response to us how best to approach him.

Certainly in Michael's case, quite apart from making his own hospital experience happier—and the importance of that cannot be minimised—to have explained things reasonably to him from the start and to have attempted to find ways of harnessing his widely ranging intelligence to some purposeful ends instead of battling against him and making him feel "talked down to" would have proved surprisingly rewarding for the busy nurse and saved, not lost, time.

It is most important also that those of us who are responsible for the care and well-being of children—and, indeed, of people of whatever age—should be able to appreciate and understand the limitations of those whose intelligence and power of understanding is below the average for their age.

It is only when we are aware of these children's limitations that we can suitably modify the demands we make on them. Because the standards set and the demands we make are normally geared to what is possible for the average child, those children of more limited intelligence are faced all through life with the stress of keeping up with a world that is too complex for them.

When we describe a child as being "below average" in intelligence we mean that his power of understanding and his pace and mode of learning is like that of a younger child. He is slower to grasp ideas and to build up experience on the basis of which he can judge and understand what is happening to him. We have seen that with the increase of knowledge and understanding of the world around him a child's confidence and sense of security also grows. Those duller children are often lacking in confidence because they do not so readily understand what is happening around them. They are bewildered and baffled by many things that present no difficulty to normal or brighter children.

These dull children also inevitably have much experience of failure.

I think most of us at some time may have had a horrible nightmare when we have seemed to spend the whole night trying to be in time for a train or to catch up to some person or other who always moved away just too quickly for us. Just when the train or the person it is so important for us to catch up with seems to be within reach off they start again and the whole miserable chase is on once more. I think that is what life must feel like always for many dull children. Fortunately for ourselves the nightmare ends when we waken. But unless these children are cared for by people who understand their limitations and can therefore modify the circumstances of their lives and the demands made on them, then their whole lives must be like a perpetual nightmare. Children, like ourselves, are very sensitive about their failures and must find some way in their behaviour of either compensating for or escaping from it.

Joan was seventeen and a half when I saw her first at an outpatients clinic of a hospital's department of psychological medicine. She was a tall, well-dressed, good looking girl but with a slightly sullen expression. She was the only child of middle class parents and she had been brought up in a very sheltered home. She had been educated at a small private day school where she had never made much progress and she left school at sixteen with only the barest smattering of knowledge of the basic subjects. She could only read the very simplest first reader—and that with difficulty—her knowledge and grasp of numbers was very rudimentary and she could not manage even very simple money sums at all. In spite of this because of her home background she spoke with a very good accent and her use of language, which she had acquired largely by imitation of the people in her home environment, gave the misleading impression that she was normally intelligent.

During the year and a half between leaving school and coming to the hospital clinic Joan had been in seven different jobs. She had started out by wanting to take up hairdressing but after a few weeks left at the firm's request because she "showed no aptitude at all for it". Then she went to help in a private day nursery near her home but again they could not keep her because, they said, "she did such stupid things". This pattern of getting a job, failing and leaving was dismally repeated throughout the whole eighteen months. Sometimes the complaint was that Joan was sullen and stupid and sometimes that she had outbursts of temper. In her last job of dressmaking she had badly hurt another girl by stabbing at her eye with a pair of scissors. This girl had teased Joan because she was so slow and got in such a muddle and Joan had been goaded beyond what she could bear.

On tests, Joan had an Intelligence Quotient of 62. That means in terms of mental age that although seventeen and a half years old she had only the capacity for understanding that we could expect of an average child of not quite ten years. Until she started work her limitations had been hidden in many ways by the protective environment of her school and home.

When her mother was told about Joan's limited mental ability and asked whether she had not noticed it before she told how slow Joan had been to learn to dress herself, how when she was sent an errand she brought the wrong things or the wrong change and how when she helped to lay the table she could never from one time to the next remember to do what she had been shown. "But," her mother added, "I thought she was being deliberately naughty and did it to annoy me".

A child whose I.Q. is 62 is very subnormal indeed; so much so that he cannot really benefit from ordinary school teaching but needs educating in what are called "Special schools for educationally sub-normal children." Joan's parents were elderly and they had no experience of other children and thus never became aware of the extent of Joan's limitations. As a consequence, she was I have no doubt, frequently punished for what seemed to them "deliberate naughtiness" when in fact her tiresome behaviour arose directly out of her inborn defect of intelligence.

Joan and Michael are extreme cases. We have seen that they could both have been helped to modify their tempestuous behaviour if the adults caring for them had understood something of their developmental needs and so tempered the pressures which their environment was making on them. Michael needed more opportunity to experiment and learn, more recognition of his ability to behave responsibly and freedom from the niggling and meaningless regulations that he found so irksome. Joan needed simpler explanations that were related for her to practical reality, more patient general handling and a relief from the pressure of being expected to achieve what was beyond her capability. Between these two extremes you will find among people in hospital many variations in the capacity to understand. Coming into the hospital is a new experience for all patients. A nurse can do much to help to lessen the strangeness and bewildering quality of this experience by helping them to understand the routine—what is happening and why it happens in that way.

This applies not only to children but to adults also. A nurse who appreciates how great the individual differences in mental ability among people can be will more easily understand why there are differences in behaviour and attitude among her various patients and be able to take their differences into account.

CHAPTER VII

The Sick Child

1. THE EMOTIONALLY DISTURBED CHILD

IN our study of the normal course of the development of healthy children we have seen that during his growth from the complete dependence of babyhood to the comparative independence of his school days, a child is bound to meet with many difficulties. However wise and understanding parents are they must inevitably make mistakes sometimes for they are only human and they too have their own problems. In any case many of the difficulties and problems of growing up can only be met and lived through by the child himself however much we may seek to help and protect him. Even the best of parents, moreover, are sometimes caught by circumstances they cannot control and, despite all their care, the child's confidence and straightforward, happy development is temporarily marred.

A child who is not developing normally and happily, whose emotional development is temporarily disturbed or out of balance, shows that he is what we might call psychologically sick by many differing symptoms depending on such factors as his age, his mental development. his personality and temperament and the kind of stresses to which he is exposed. He may suffer from night terrors and fears; he may be excessively shy; he may suck his thumb or bite his nails; he may lie and steal; he may be destructive; or he may be unable to play normally with other children. He may be unduly late in learning to talk or he may not be able to learn to read and keep up with school work even although he is as intelligent as the other children in his group.

These are just a few of the ways by which a child may show that the normal, happy course of his development is disturbed and that he is, at any rate temporarily, emotionally maladjusted.

All children at times have emotional troubles. These troubles are part of the business of growing up. Indeed in the pre-school years emotional troubles for the child are so usual as to be regarded as almost 'normal'. But the healthily developing child, basically secure in his good home and supported during times of difficulty by the loving care of understanding parents, works through his problems.

Those whose job it is to care for children need to be able to distinguish what might be described as symptoms of 'normal' emotional stress and those that point to more serious psychological illness. To take a simple example, temper tantrums, distressing as they are, are a normal symptom of emotional stress in a child of two or three years old. But if we find a much older child, for example a child of eight or nine, still having temper tantrums we know that he is emotionally a very sick child indeed and that he probably needs specialised help to overcome his difficulties. Just as in physical development, there are many temporary upsets during the period of childhood that any sensible mother can deal with without calling in the help of a doctor. When a child has a stomach upset and is sick we know that it is so common in childhood as to be, as it were, a 'normal' symptom of temporary upset and we know what to do to help the child to recover. But if the sickness persists and is accompanied by a great deal of pain then it is part of the good mother's job to be able to recognise that the symptoms may indicate a more serious condition that demands the specialised help of a skilled physician.

Similarly if we know what to expect of a child during the ordinary course of development we can distinguish between 'normal' symptoms of temporary emotional stress and more serious symptoms which point to the child's need for the kind of specialised help given in Child Guidance clinics.

Most children show that they are undergoing extra emotional stress by difficult, unsettled behaviour of some kind or another. It is important to try to recognise this tiresome behaviour as a child's appeal for help rather than deliberate naughtiness.

When a child's confidence in himself has been shaken, so that he feels insecure, bewildered and afraid, he often shows it in ways that are irritating and annoying to grown-ups. It is at times like this that he needs extra comfort and support. Unless we understand the kind of problems and difficulties which children have to meet in the course of growing up it is easy to confuse symptoms of emotional stress with deliberate misbehaviour and, by scolding and punishing the child, fail to meet his need for reassurance and help. It is often easier to help a child who is physically sick because it is so much easier to recognise that he is ill. If he has a cold or is sick we do not scold him but rather do all that we can to get him well again. And if we can recognise that a great deal of unsettled behaviour in children is a symptom of emotional ill-health, quite as real and damaging to the child's total development as physical ill-health, and can keep our patience and give the child the extra reassurance and support that he so urgently needs, his own recuperative powers will often do the rest of what is needed to restore his emotional adjustment.

Children who are suffering from emotional disturbance show it in many different ways. In some children it finds expression in excessively angry, aggressive behaviour. They have violent temper tantrums, they scream, they scratch and bite and attack other children or they are wantonly destructive of their own or other people's possessions. They tear their clothes or bed linen, damage toys, tear up books, knock down the brick towers or sand castles made by other children. The destructive child finds an outlet for his aggressive feelings by attacking objects in the external world. Such behaviour in children is stimulated by deep feelings of hatred and jealousy, probably towards their own parents, with which they have not found any way of coming to terms and which they cannot express more directly against their real parents. This kind of disturbed behaviour is more common in the younger pre-school child but sometimes older children return to it when they are deeply upset in any way. During the war I had a little boy billeted with me. Tommy was seven and a half when I took him. He had been in six different homes and had then been put into a hostel for unbilletable children. But he created such problems for the hostel that I decided to take him home with me.

The first night after he was tucked up in bed and apparently happily settled for sleep he produced a pair of scissors and cut his blankets into innumerable little pieces. He had been moved from his last billet at the request of a very motherly country woman. She had been warned that Tommy was difficult and destructive and that five other mothers in the village had asked for him to be moved but had thought that she could, as she put it, "get round" any child. It was more than she could bear, however, when she saw her very best table cloth cut into ribbons and her lovely silk tea cosy smouldering on the fire. Tommy was indeed a very deeply disturbed and anxious child. He badly wanted to be loved and accepted in his billet but it seemed as if he had to try out each foster-mother by being bad and destructive. And unfortunately for him he had proved to himself six times that he was too bad to be accepted.

My home and possessions had to suffer a good deal of destruction, even though I tried hard to prevent him from using scissors and knives and destructive weapons, before he could convince himself that although I would not let him spoil and break up everything I still wanted to keep him and that I would not take revenge on him for his destructiveness by severe punishments.

Tommy was psychologically a very sick child indeed. His difficulties were too great to be overcome simply by giving him a consistently friendly and tolerant environment. But a stable foster-home background provided the necessary co-operation for specialised treatment at a Child Guidance clinic to prove capable of straightening out his problems.

Some children show their anxiety in an entirely different way. They are excessively shy, dreamy and withdrawn. These children seem to be so afraid of their real world that they retreat into a phantasy world of their own imagining. They become inactive and solitary. They often do badly at school because they are inattentive. They cannot give their minds to real problems immediately to hand because their thoughts are taken up with inner problems and day-dreams of their own. Often these children are not recognised as 'problem' children because they are not a nuisance in the way that the angry, aggressive child is a nuisance. But their emotional disturbance can be quite as serious and just as damaging to their total healthy growth.

Habit disorders of many different kinds are all expressions of some inner need that is unsatisfied or a reaction to some form of stress or anxiety.

It is perhaps easiest to understand and therefore be more able to tolerate the emotionally disturbed child if we try to relate the kind of symptoms that he shows to the level of development of which they are a characteristic expression.

Most of the emotional disorder that occurs during late infancy and the early pre-school years arises from difficulties in the child's feeling relationships, primarily with his mother. We have already seen that the infant's first need is the satisfaction of the primitive impulses for food and warmth and comfort. An infant finds satisfaction for these early needs partly from his own mother and partly from his own body. When the relationship between the mother and the child is not wholly satisfactory the child turns to his own body for comfort. Thumb-sucking, rocking and a little later, masturbating are all characteristic habits whereby the child seeks for more pleasurable sensations.

Feeding difficulties are a common type of difficulty in infancy and early childhood. When we remember that food and the giver of food are very much identified for the child during his first year and that his love for his mother grows out of his love for the comfort that she provides for him, it is not surprising that many disturbances in the child-mother relationship can easily find expression in difficulties regarding food. It is a well-founded observation that children who are faddy and difficult over eating at home often present no feeding difficulties at all when they have their meals with other children, for example in a Nursery School. Although they outgrow these difficulties, for many people the idea of food and mother remain bound together in their minds and influences often quite unreasonably their reaction to food throughout their lives.

During the last war many country mothers who took in evacuee children from the towns and had looked forward with pleasure and pride to giving them the enjoyment of good wholesome country food were bitterly disappointed that some of the very poor town children still hankered for the "pennorth of chips" put before them in the rough and ready way of their slum homes. I came to know some of these children well and it was often clear that it seemed to them almost an act of disloyalty to the mother they loved to enjoy meals so different from those it had seemed good to her to provide. This kind of unconscious relating of feelings about food and feelings about people often lasts long past childhood. After all a song that was very popular among young servicemen began

"Ma, I miss your apple pie,
Ma, I miss your stew" . . .

and ended

"Ma I miss you too."

Children of two to three years frequently show angry, aggressive behaviour which finds its expression in temper tantrums, screaming and destructiveness. This again, is understandable when we remind ourselves of what problems arise for the child out of his developmental experiences. Although he is beginning to feel urged by his inner growth to strive towards greater independence of achievement he is constantly frustrated by his own limitations and reminded of his own inadequacy and littleness, and his own control is still weak. It is not surprising therefore that when the demands life makes on him becomes too great for him his control breaks down and he finds an outlet for his anger and feelings of frustration by screaming and temper tantrums. As children develop more skill and mastery over their material world and wider understanding of it their sense of proportion grows and the number and intensity of aggressive outbursts decreases.

Other difficulties characteristically occurring during the early years of childhood are difficulties in bowel and bladder control, night terrors and fears of being left alone in the dark. Children of two to four years often develop sudden and what appears to the grown-up person, quite unreasoning fears or phobias.

From about five years of age the child's emotional life becomes for him steadily more manageable and he consequently becomes more stable and fewer difficulties occur. The difficulties so characteristic of the earlier period when the child had so many problems to resolve and while his feeling relationships with his parents and intimate family circle still played so large a part in his total experience gradually disappear. The child who still has problems of adjustment shows them more characteristically in anti-social behaviour. He expresses defiance and stubbornness through obstinacy and indifference rather than by tempers and screaming. Feeding difficulties disappear and are often replaced by enuresis.

Anti-social behaviour in the form of mild delinquencies such as stealing and truanting occur in the school-age period of 7 to 11 years. But generally with the child who is developing normally there is much less evidence of emotional stress during this period of childhood.

In periods of crisis, such as, for example, that experienced by the child at the birth of a baby in his family, this intensity of anxiety and rivalry finds expression in a regression to an earlier level of development. At times like this an older child may show his stress in symptoms which relate to a much earlier phase of development. Even for an adult, intense anxiety can revive patterns of behaviour and attitudes long since out-grown. We shall refer to this again when we come to consider adult patients in hospital and the problems related to them. But meanwhile let us turn our attention to the sick child in hospital.

II. THE SICK CHILD IN HOSPITAL

Because emotional stress, fear, anxiety and insecurity in children find their expression in unsettled behaviour of one kind or another nurses caring for sick children in hospital will inevitably meet with a good deal of trying behaviour in their young patients.

Children in hospital are suffering from a dual stress.

1. Children are taken into hospital when they are physically very sick—too sick to be nursed in their own homes. In describing the course of development of the human being from infancy through childhood I have emphasised the fact that physical, mental and emotional growth are so inextricably interwoven that truly healthy development depends on total well-being in all its aspects. A child who is physically sick is inevitably to some extent emotionally sick also because his total well-being is thrown out of balance. This of course is true of all sick people but it is particularly evident in children because their

security is not so firmly based and they are still at an immature stage of growth when their sense of security is to a greater or less extent dependent on their good relationship with the people who care for them and who form the known background of their lives.

Those of you who have had anything to do with sick children in their own homes will know how extra difficult, extra fretful and demanding they are at such times. The feeling of 'dis-ease', the feeling of frustration because they cannot manage to do the things they want to do and can normally do, in itself arouses anxiety. You will often hear a mother say "My Billy is so peevish and cross that I'm sure he must be sickening for something".

Because a characteristic mode of reacting to illness in grown-ups as well as children is to regress to an earlier pattern of behaviour children who are sick usually become extra demanding of the mother's time and attention. A child who in his normal behaviour is sturdy and independent, eager to go out and play with other children, will become afraid to let his mother out of his sight and want her to stay near him all through his waking hours. In this demand for extra mothering it is as if the child unconsciously feels that by retreating to an earlier phase of development he will recapture some of the feeling of security that his closeness to his mother and greater dependence on her gave. Just because he is ill, therefore, he is undergoing psychological stress also.

2. At this time when the child's illness is upsetting the even balance of his emotional development and arousing in him feelings of anxiety which make him cry out for extra mothering, he is, because of the seriousness of his physical illness, taken into hospital. Just at the time, therefore, when he has to meet the stresses created for him by being physically sick he has the added stress of having

to adapt to a sudden and complete break in the continuity of his environment and cope with the anxiety inevitably aroused by being cared for by strangers instead of by his own parents whom he knows and trusts.

During recent years a considerable body of evidence has been accumulated from psychological research regarding the effect of the separation of the young child from his parents during the early years of growth. These research studies all emphasise the fact that the most important developmental need of the young child is the constant, steady, loving care that is given him by his mother or mother substitute. During infancy he needs to be able to form a relationship with *one* clearly identified person—that is his mother or one person who has taken the place of his real mother. Dr. Bowlby has brought together all these different research studies in his report for the World Health Organisation. Although a great deal of further study remains to be done in this field the accumulated evidence from research studies up to date suggests that after the fifth or sixth month of life the infant is able to extend his interest and feeling for people more widely and comes to know and enjoy his father and, later, his brothers and sisters and other people who form a familiar part of his intimate world. But if his growth and development is to continue satisfactorily he needs his mother as an ever-present companion up to the time when he is about three years old.

Gradually he begins to be able to maintain his relationship with his mother even when she is absent but until he is about five years old he cannot keep alive his relationship with her if he is separated from her for more than a few days or weeks at most.

These age norms vary widely among individual children according to their maturity of development. But there is fairly clear evidence that unless the child is able to establish these relationships during early childhood the development of his mind and feelings is vitally impaired and it is doubtful whether the damage suffered can ever really be made good. To quote Dr. Bowlby, "The unfolding of the child's self and conscience can only go on satisfactorily when his first human relationships are continuous and happy."

These research findings place on nurses a very great responsibility for during a period of illness in hospital a young child is deprived of one of his most vital needs—loving care by his own mother. The younger the child, the more serious can be the effects of this separation.

Eminent children's doctors in many countries have from their own observations become increasingly aware of the serious effects of separation of a young child from his mother during illness and in some of the most modern children's hospitals arrangements are now made for mothers of young children to stay in hospital and share in the nursing care of their sick children. The treatment of children in the hospitals where this arrangement can be carried out has proved so successful that there can be little doubt that sick children need not only skilled nursing but also continuity of mothering for their satisfactory recovery.

In the majority of children's hospitals, however, arrangements whereby the mother can stay with and share in the nursing care of her child during his illness are not possible. In these hospitals, therefore, it is an essential part of good nursing to satisfy for the child this need for mothering as far as possible.

I want to discuss now some of the ways in which nurses can lessen for children the severity of the effects of this separation and reduce the stresses which coming into hospital creates for the child.

Of course there are some things that lie outside the control of the individual nurse because they are part of the general policy of the hospital. One of the most important of these is the question of allowing parents to visit the child in hospital frequently. There are even yet in this country a few children's hospitals where no visiting is allowed at all. It has been argued that because children are upset and cry each time their parents leave after visiting them it is better not to expose them to this repeated upset. Psychologists, however, are agreed that regular visiting by the parents not only increases the child's happiness and feeling of security while he is in hospital but it also helps to maintain for him the continuity of his experience. This makes it easier for him to return home, when the time comes, with much less emotional upheaval than he would experience if he had not been helped by his parents' visits, and in other ways, to keep alive in his mind the idea of his place in his real home.

When the mother is allowed to pop in frequently and informally to see her child his distress when she leaves gradually diminishes for he begins to know by the experience of her coming and going that he has not completely lost her. Even if he is upset when she leaves him it is better for him to cry over this real sorrow and turn to the nurse for comfort than to lie fretting and bewildered by the feeling of a permanent loss of a mother who never comes at all. One of the things most difficult for young children to grasp is the concept of time. There are still very many hospitals where visiting of children is only allowed once or sometimes twice a week. This length of time between visits is too great for a young child to conceive and the waiting period must seem quite endless.

Although the decision as to how frequently parents should be allowed to visit their children in hospital lies outside the young nurse's control there are many ways by which a nurse who understands and appreciates the child's psychological needs can lessen the severity of the emotional injury that can result from separation from parents during a period of illness in hospital.

A child's emotional security grows out of the assurance that he is loved and wanted because he is a worth-while person who merits love and regard. I think it is true to say of any child who is emotionally disturbed that at the core of his problem is the feeling, whether based on something real or only imaginary, that he has lost the assurance of his own value. We have seen that this feeling of security on which sound mental health is founded comes in the first place from the good relation between a young child and his mother. It grows out of her love and her care for him and the orderly and thoughtful way in which she looks after him and plans for him until he has developed far enough to begin to manage things for himself and act independently of her. It is the steady and loving care of his parents for him in a stable home where circumstances do not change too sharply or too suddenly for the child to be able to understand and adjust himself to them that builds up for him this feeling of being secure in a world in which he is loved and has a place. He feels safe because there are always loving and stable adults who help to keep his background of experience steady. Even if his own primitive impulses and emotions threaten to get the better of him there is always Mummy or Daddy to help to keep things in control for him. And they are people who can go on loving him even if the bad in him gets the mastery for a time. They are people who can reassure him and build up his confidence in his own maturity.

Coming into hospital constitutes a very sharp change in the circumstances of a child's life. And just when he is suddenly robbed of all that is familiar in his way of life —and this in itself is very alarming and unsettling particularly for a young child—so that he needs his parents most of all he has to do without them.

Although obviously the nurse cannot replace the child's mother she can provide for the child some of the essential qualities of good mothering and in this way give him a sense of continuity in his emotional experience so that the change from home to hospital is not so great. By being patient, tolerant and, most important of all, consistent in her ways with him, she can show the child that in hospital as well as at home he is cared for by people who have *good feeling* towards him. The child is greatly helped by having people to care for him who are reliable in their friendliness towards him. That is why children can best be helped by people who are themselves stable and mature. A person who is unhappy or disturbed in her own life must be sufficiently mature not to 'take it out of' the children in her care because she herself is unhappy. One of the things that cuts sharply at the root of a child's security is to be cared for by an adult who is moody and changeable. Similarly dis-harmony between grown-ups who are caring for a child is most distressing to the child. Whatever her own personal feelings and problems may be a nurse should for this reason endeavour to keep the reliability of her feeling towards her patient separate and intact.

It is not always easy to maintain this good feeling if the child's anxiety shows itself in troublesome behaviour as it so frequently does. Perhaps it is a help if we can carry in our minds some general principles for handling a disturbed child whatever is the symptom by which he shows it.

It is important that we should recognise that the tiresome behaviour, be it soiling or wetting or thumb sucking or general fretfulness, is a symptom and that we do not help by attacking the symptom directly. The tiresome behaviour will disappear when the reason for it has gone. We can, of course, stop a great deal of tiresome behaviour by force, by threats or by fear. But unless the real reason for it has gone the anxiety and the emotional stress of which such behaviour is an expression will show itself in some other way. If we want to stop the steam from coming out of the spout of the kettle we do not bung up the spout because we know that the steam will find another way to get out. To stop it we must take the kettle off the heat and stop the water from boiling. We can stop a child from sucking his thumb by putting his arm in splints so that he cannot get his thumb to his mouth or we can punish him so severely that the fear of the punishment is greater than the comfort he gets from sucking his thumb. But in neither of these ways will we have resolved the need for comfort and reassurance of which his thumb-sucking is the expression.

We must remember also that it is not much use asking a child why he does these things. Most of the difficulties which find expression in these ways are not at a conscious level and the child himself does not know "Why?"

We must guard therefore against making the child feel still more guilty or ashamed of his behaviour. Even when it is necessary to restrain him from what he is doing we must try to convey that while we cannot allow him to behave in that way we are still 'on the child's side' in the sense that we are giving him our support in overcoming his difficulties. In this way and by the constancy of our friendliness towards him we can convey to the child that although we may dislike, and will not allow, his behaviour at a particular time our basic good feeling for him remains unshaken.

This is particularly necessary when a child's anxiety expresses itself in temper tantrums or violent outbursts of destructiveness or anger. A temper tantrum is a most distressing symptom to deal with and it is also a very terrifying experience for the child himself because for the time being he is completely at the mercy of all the forces of aggression and anger that he so greatly fears within himself. At times like these the child needs restraint that is firm while remaining kind. He needs to feel that while we cannot allow him to attack other children or attack us we are not angry with him. He is helped by the feeling that we are strong enough and controlled enough to support him and prevent his anger from being too damaging until he can regain his own control. At times like this it is often necessary to take the child away from other children but he should not be shut away by himself and left to deal with this anger alone. It is easier to remain patient and tolerant if we remind ourselves that we are dealing not merely with a naughty child but with one who is in great need of our support and help.

Ronald was a boy of nine whom I came to know well during his time in hospital and for some years afterwards. He had had a mastoid operation and had suffered great pain. Whenever the time came for a dressing he was terrified and resisted it with all his might. He screamed and kicked and worked himself up into a panic and rage that was quite distressing to see. It would have been easy to regard this boy—nine years, old—as a naughty, bad-tempered cry-baby. He could probably have been controlled by severity, by putting him in a room alone, or by punishing him for these outbursts. But this would only have increased his anxiety by deepening his sense of rejection and would have delayed his recovery.

Fortunately he came under the care of a nurse of great experience who was able to recognise that apart from the mastoid operation he was an extremely emotionally sick child. I noted her treatment of him with great interest. It was so psychologically *right* that it is, I think, worth while recording in some detail.

She made it her business to find time to give him what has been so aptly described as "slow-handed" care. She never rushed him but was always patient in her attitude to him. However busy she really was she never appeared to be in such a hurry that she had not time for him.

She never said a lot of unnecessary "Don'ts" but was quite firm and consistent in seeing that the rules and restrictions that were really necessary were always kept.

When he asked a question she treated it sensibly and tried to answer it simply and at his level of understanding. But she always answered it truthfully. She often had to answer his questionings by saying, "Yes, this *will* hurt." But she never left it like that. She always went on to explain why it was necessary to do this thing that would hurt him. She tried to cut through his fear and apprehension by explaining at a simple level the things that happened to him. Gradually she built up for him a great feeling of their partnership in working together to get him well again.

As he began to recover she did her best to provide him with suitable occupations and interests. Knowing that there had been much in his experience that he needed to sort over in his mind and that he could probably do this best through the medium of imaginative play she made available to him the kind of toys and material most suitable for this kind of play. She gathered up a box of odds and ends, a family of small dolls, a set of nurse and doctor dolls, toy furniture, little cups and spoons and bottles, some animals domestic and wild, a few dinky toy motors, aeroplanes and trains, some bricks and bits of things that could be used to set a scene and made to fit in, in varying ways, with his imaginings. Although she made these readily available should he want them she did not thrust them at him nor seem to be disappointed when he occupied himself quite differently or used toys with quite a different purpose from those they were intended for.

He often played games in which frightening things happened to a child in hospital and in his games he frequently made the nurse and the doctor and his own parents behave in ways that made them seem like ogres or cruel monsters. But although Ronald's phantasy play was often very babyish for a boy of nine she never ridiculed it or tried to direct it, guessing that it was somehow satisfying a very real need by allowing him to work out his problems and thus regain his emotional adjustment.

Because his play was so very real to him she tried to avoid having to interrupt it too suddenly and when the time was approaching when it would have to be interrupted and the toys cleared away, carefully gave him some warning beforehand. She used to tell him what was going to happen next in the ward and why, therefore, his toys would have to be packed up and his bed made tidy and would explain what she would be doing before she came to tidy him up so that he would have time to bring that imaginative play to a close.

She always listened carefully when Ronnie talked about his parents, his home, and his school and soon learned that Ronnie was very worried about school and about missing his "Sums and Reading" lessons. It was clear from his talk that he had found school work hard enough to cope with before his illness and was worrying a great deal about what it would be like for him when he went back to school.

An educational psychologist part of whose job was to sort out these school difficulties for a sick child was attached to the staff of the Child Guidance clinic in the hospital. The nurse therefore reported Ronnie's school difficulties through the proper channels and the psychologist was able to help Ronnie with some of his school learning problems while he was convalescing and, by visiting the school and explaining about his illness and his difficulties and consequent worries to his teachers, to make his return to school much less difficult than it might otherwise have been.

If you look back over the things that this nurse did for Ronnie and her attitude to him you will see that she behaved towards him very much in the way that any good mother would. Because she appreciated the stress that Ronnie was experiencing and the extent of his insecurity she was able to tolerate his trying behaviour with the same patience that any good mother has for her needy child. But—and this is very important—she never tried to replace his own mother in his affections. On the contrary, I noticed that she tried in innumerable ways to help Ronnie to keep alive his feeling for his own mother.

Ronnie's problems had by no means started with his arrival in hospital. He had in fact, as the nurse had instinctively recognised, been a very difficult and disturbed child long before this illness. It is reasonable to suppose that in his moments of anger he must have had very hateful and destructive feelings towards his parents. As we have seen earlier a young child cannot easily distinguish between absence and death. And for this reason a long separation from his mother arouses in a child vaguely anxious feelings that he has lost her for ever and that perhaps he himself has brought this about.

Emotionally Ronald was far below the normal developmental level of a healthy nine-year old. When he was left in hospital without his mother, and, as was found out later, with no truthful explanation of what was about to happen to him, he suffered, as his imaginative play later showed, quite frightening feelings of guilt that his mother was dead and that he himself had destroyed her by his angry thoughts. When this nurse first saw Ronnie and said, "Hello, I know you, you're called Ronnie, aren't you?" he gave that reply which so many children in hospital give, "Yes, I *am* called Ronnie and I *have* got a Mum and a Dad."

All through his time in hospital Ronnie gave this same reply to every stranger who greeted him. It seemed as though he needed to reassure himself constantly on that subject. Recognising this the nurse helped him greatly by talking about his "Mum and Dad" and by encouraging him to talk about them to her. She saved anything that he had done, his little pictures and drawings and things he made, so that he could show them to his mother when she visited him and obviously did everything she could to keep alive and foster the bond that was between them. I imagine she cannot always have found this easy because Ronnie's mother was in fact a rather stupid person who in many ways undid the good things that had been done for Ronnie while he was in hospital. But I saw that she tried hard never to allow Ronnie, either by criticising his Mother in his hearing or by her attitude to her when she visited him, to sense this feeling, appreciating that his relationship with his mother was the most important bond in his childhood and knowing from her long experience that it was a part of good nursing to help to keep this relationship intact despite the inevitable separation which being in hospital had caused.

Most children, of course, are much more stable than Ronnie was. And in any case they would not necessarily show their anxiety in the same ways. But I have dealt in some detail with the case of Ronnie and one nurse's way of handling him because it seems to me to indicate the main basic psychological principles that hold good for the nursing of all sick children.

III. PSYCHOLOGICAL PROBLEMS OF PHYSICALLY HANDICAPPED CHILDREN

Physical handicaps take many different forms and consequently create differing kinds of deprivation for those who suffer under them. If these children are to be cared for adequately their difficulties need to be understood and recognised. The nature and also the extent of the deprivation from which physically handicapped children suffer varies with each individual child. It may however be useful briefly to point out some of the main kinds of deprivation and the kind of psychological problems to which they give rise, although the discussion of this vast field in any detail lies outside the scope of this book.

In considering the deprivations of the disabled child it cannot be too strongly emphasised that no handicap or deprivation which results from disability can be defined, or separated in its effects, from the total personality. It impinges on the whole growth and development and affects it in limitless directions.

For a child who cannot hear or a child who cannot see, one important channel for receiving experience from the outside world is blocked for him. Serious as is the deprivation of the blind child that of the totally deaf child is even greater. Because of his deafness, unless it is detected early and he is specially taught, he cannot hear speech and he cannot use words either as a means of communication with other people or as a tool of thought. If he cannot use words in his thinking, the range of his thought and consequently the opportunities necessary for the full development of his intelligence are very much restricted. His emotional and social growth is also limited because speech is such a necessary link in human relationships.

For such children not only is their capacity to receive experiences from the outside world affected but their ability to communicate with other people in their world is also limited.

This is the case to an even more severe degree for children, such as those suffering from cerebral palsy, whose handicap affects both motor and sensory capacities. For many such children the power to communicate their thoughts to others by means of speech, writing and movement are, in varying degrees according to the extent of the brain damage, blocked, even though their powers of reasoning and thought may be relatively unimpaired. In the past many of these children were wrongly judged to be feeble-minded.

Perhaps one of the clearest examples of the way in which physical health and well-being are bound up with the healthy development of mind and feelings—in short, with total growth—can be seen in the problems of behaviour and learning with which many brain-damaged children are faced. Because they suffer frequently from difficulties of perception, they cannot easily organise their world into a meaningful pattern. They cannot learn as quickly as normally developing children do to pick out essential from non-essential perceptions. Because their world is such a confusing and dis-organised place for them, many brain damaged children are extremely distractible and lacking in control. Nigel is a seven-year old spastic boy whom I saw recently for an assessment of his intelligence. His physical disability was hardly noticeable and to anyone who was not aware of it he could only appear to be a restless, uncontrolled and clumsy child. It was almost impossible to hold his interest for more than a few minutes at a time and in between he would run round the room, clumsily banging into furniture as he went. He needed to be guarded from falling into the fire or tumbling over the toys on the floor. He behaved in this way not because he was deliberately careless and troublesome but because the brain damage he had suffered made it difficult for him to judge the distances between objects in order that his perceptions could guide his movements as would be the case for a normally healthy seven-year old child. This difficulty in patterning his world and in distinguishing between objects that are near and those that are further away make the world a confusing place for Nigel. This has created for him an anxiety to which he can only respond by restless, impulsive behaviour.

All these children, as well as many others such as diabetics and epileptic children, are, by reason of their handicap, separated and different from normally healthy children and in consequence they all suffer from extra frustrations. In varying ways the opportunities for normal emotional development and expression are denied them.

We have already seen what a valuable outlet and 'safety-valve' as well as a means of learning, play provides for the growing child. For many handicapped children, cut off as they are from so many normal experiences, the imaginative content of their play is very limited. Children whose handicap affects their movement are deprived also of all the stimulating experiences that come through active play. It is not surprising that most of these children, because their modes of expression and their emotional outlets are very limited, find what appear to be very uncontrolled ways of expression when normal outlets such as speech are not possible for them. We must remember that these children are constantly experiencing situations that arouse in them very great feelings of frustration—feelings much more intense than a normally healthy child is ever required to bear. And because of their deprivations they have never had the same chance as the normal child of building up a firm sense of security. It is not surprising, therefore, they are often less stable.

In their desire to compensate to them for what they are missing mothers of handicapped children tend to over-protect them and guard them from activity and experiences which are a necessary part of learning to grow up. Children who have been over-protected in this way are often very difficult to console or to help to become adjusted to hospital life and to the separation from their own mothers. While avoiding over-protecting them or subjecting them to the humiliating effects of pity, we must always try to retain an awareness of the psychological effects on all handicapped children of their extra difficulties and in our care for them try to anticipate their extra needs, needs which they themselves often cannot find a way to express.

CHAPTER VIII

Adolescence

THE period which we are now about to consider represents the final stage in the growth towards adulthood. It covers roughly the time from about twelve years old for girls, usually somewhat later for boys' to the late teens or early twenties—that is the 'teen-age' period. It can be divided into two fairly clearly defined phases. There is the early adolescent period which is marked by the onset of puberty when the physical changes towards manhood and womanhood take place and the physical readiness for sexual maturity is achieved. This is followed by a period of emotional adjustment to the extensive physical changes that have taken place.

In our study of the development of the human being through infancy and childhood we have seen that all growth is a continuous process and the way in which a person meets and adjusts himself to each changing phase and the new demands that it makes on him depends on the extent to which his earlier development has been smooth and satisfactory. We have seen also how closely the physical, mental and emotional aspects of growth and well-being are interwoven. This again is seen most strikingly during adolescence.

The period of late childhood, immediately preceding the changes that occur in adolescence, is, as we have seen, a time of comparative stability. During this period the child as a result of his widening interests in the real world and the satisfactions of active comradeship with other children, is able to turn away from inner phantasy and make-believe and to become less involved emotionally with his own family. The conflicts and turbulence of early childhood, even if not wholly resolved, are for the time being repressed and 'latent'. Indeed the psychological term for this period is the 'latency period'.

In contrast with the steady, even growth of the latency period, rapid physical changes usher in the beginning of adolescence and cause big new pressures to be placed on the young person's emotional adjustment. If emotional conflicts have not been resolved during the stage of development to which they properly belonged they tend to arise again in adolescence with overwhelming force.

In many ways this final stage of growth to manhood or womanhood resembles in its stresses and turbulence the period of early childhood and much of its difficulty can best be understood by relating it to what has gone before. If a child has not been able to work through his feelings of love, hate and rivalry towards his parents and brothers and sisters and come to terms with inevitable feelings of jealousy during the early childhood years this final phase of growth towards emotional independence and maturity is not likely to be easy. The extent to which a young person will be able to make satisfactory relationships during adolescence, and later as an adult, depends on the degree to which he has been able in early childhood to experience warm and loving relationships with his mother and father and with the important adults who then made up his world.

Winnicott and Britton, who were responsible for one county's hostels for difficult and unbilletable evacuees during the last war, have aptly described these early needs as "primary home experiences". The meaning of this has been so well expressed by them that I should like to quote it in full: "By a primary home experience is meant experience of an environment adapted to the special needs of the infant and the little child, without which the foundations of mental health cannot be laid down. Without someone specifically orientated to his needs the infant cannot find a working relation to external reality. Without someone to give satisfactory instinctual gratifications the infant cannot find his body, nor can he develop an integrated personality. Without one person to love and to hate he cannot come to know that it is the same person that he loves and hates and so cannot find his sense of guilt and his desire to repair and restore. Without a limited human and physical environment that he can know he cannot find out the extent to which his aggressive ideas actually fail to destroy and so cannot sort out the difference between phantasy and fact. Without a father and a mother who are together and who take joint responsibility for him, he cannot find and express his urge to separate them, nor experience relief at failing to do so. The emotional development of the first years is complex and cannot be skipped over and every infant absolutely needs a certain degree of favourable environment if he is to negotiate the essential first stages of this development."

The pattern of the feeling relationships with other people that the adolescent is able to form is based on the patterns of feeling laid down in the course of these primary experiences.

Working in psychological clinics with adolescents who have been brought up in institutions or who have for some reason or other suffered severe breaks in the continuity of their relationships in childhood one is struck by certain characteristics which occur so frequently as to seem almost typical. Chief among these is their difficulty in making any permanent friendships or in forming anything but superficial relationships with other people.

Even the feelings and attitudes of young people from normal, happy homes are coloured to a great extent as they grow up by their early attitudes to their own parents. Let me give a very simple example. A young nurse of my acquaintance who had always had conflict with her own very domineering mother—a conflict which she had never resolved—found it difficult to accept female authority of any kind. As a consequence when she chose nursing as a career she found herself faced again and again with the sort of situation she had found so intolerable at home and for a time her reaction to this seemed likely to wreck her nursing career. Only very gradually and with a good deal of help from older people was she able to develop sufficient insight into her feelings of defiance and antagonism to be able to grapple with them. But she had to travel a long and stormy journey through her training years before she was able to come to terms with her rebellious feelings and accept the position of having other women in authority over her.

Let us consider now what are the stresses which make this adolescent period difficult. We will briefly consider first the changes caused by physical growth.

The onset of adolescence is usually characterised by greatly accelerated growth both in height and weight. This increase in height and weight is accompanied by changes in the internal organs of the body which are related to variations in the functioning of the endocrine glands. Glands which regulate the development of sex characteristics come into action and by the end of puberty the physical capacity for adult sexual experience and the powers of reproduction are achieved. With this go alterations in the bodily structure and appearance: the child is changing into the adult.

The change is in many ways much sharper and, because of the beginning of menstruation, much more clearly defined for the girl than for the boy. During this period of very rapid growth there are often, also, many unevennesses of development which frequently cause quite considerable anxiety and mental discomfort to the young person who experiences them. For example girls in their early teens very often put on an excess of fat due to dysfunction of the pituitary gland. Or again, muscular tissues and bones do not grow at an even rate. Consequently the young person has difficulty in muscular co-ordination and control and is temporarily clumsy and awkward in his movements. This disharmony of functioning which occurs during these sharp physiological changes can be a source of real worry and anxiety to young people. The normal physical changes which distinguish their sex are also frequently at first a source of great embarrassment. This is often made more difficult for some young people because of the wide variations in the ages at which these changes occur. A girl may begin to menstruate or a boy's voice may break one or even two years before this happens to their friends in the same group. And some young people feel isolated and 'different' on this account.

Consciousness of the physical changes that are taking place, the temporary loss of control and the upsurge of emotional forces which the growth towards sexual maturity arouses all have their effect on psychological development. For this process of becoming grown up is not just physical maturation only but the maturing of the total personality, the movement from childhood to adulthood.

Early adolescence not only marks the final phase of physical growth and maturing but is also a time of intellectual change. The ability to reason in words and with it the power of abstract thought develops. The young person becomes much more interested in ideas than, as during childhood, in factual information. The upper limit of intelligence is reached during adolescence. This of course does not mean that after that time a person will learn no more. He will go on through adult life gathering more knowledge and more experience. But his intellectual capacity will not increase further.

Growth during adolescence is not confined to physical growth and the maturing of the sex organs; nor does the maturing of mental capacity complete the growing up process. The period of adolescence is the time during which the young person achieves the final stage in his growth towards emotional independence of his family.

In our study of the development of human behaviour we have seen that it is characteristic at all stages of growth for a person in times of stress to revert to less mature phases of development. We saw how a little child who had seemed so sturdy and independent would, on the arrival of a new baby into his home, suck his thumb again and wet his bed. It is as if he could not face the sharpness of the change in his circumstances and he did not want to be pushed into independence too quickly. The adolescent is faced with very sharp changes in the circumstances of his life. Physical maturing and with it the urge to grow up often seems to happen very quickly. It is not surprising, therefore, that one very common characteristic of the adolescent period is the swing in mood and attitude that is constantly occurring. The young person wants to grow up but he is torn between the desire to be grown up and independent and the regrets and fears aroused in leaving childhood behind. Parents and, indeed, all adults who have to do with adolescents must be prepared to find their behaviour and attitudes at times seemingly incalculable.

Sometimes they are defiant and irritated by authority, insistent on being left alone to plan for themselves and manage their own affairs. They adopt a reserve towards grown-ups and they guard their thoughts and plans and feelings from the inquisitive eye of parents and other adults. They escape into a world of their own imagining and indulge again in phantasy.

Then suddenly, without, as it seems to the bewildered parent, any observable reason, they regress to the dependency of childhood. They cannot make up their minds about things or reach a decision, they want help and adult companionship again. And the parents who have been trying hard to adjust themselves to the fact that their child has grown up and no longer needs them, find themselves once more with a needy child making great demands. This kind of regression in behaviour is an indication of the emotional conflict which the young person is undergoing. He has a healthy urge to grow up but growing up and becoming truly independent means accepting responsibilities and facing an inevitable aloneness. The young person cannot make this journey at an even pace but needs at times to retreat and experience again the reassurance and sense of dependence that belongs to the younger child.

Unevenness of progress marks adolescence in every aspect of development. In this time of sharp physical change, the young person swings between bursts of physical energy and periods of great lassitude and fatigue.

In mood also there is no middle way and the adolescent

swings between elation and despair. Similarly, their intellectual judgments tend to be 'all-or-none': it is common for adolescents to see things in terms of black and white. A thing is entirely good or entirely bad in their judgment of it and they cannot compromise. This is perhaps because they have as yet very little background of experience against which to modify their opinions. They are, however, eager to enquire into the meaning and purpose of life and are particularly concerned to understand the part they themselves should play in it. It is at this time too that they become more vividly aware of themselves and conscious of their own individuality. Until the young person has had time to develop sufficient integration within himself he tends often to be gauche, self-conscious and acutely embarrassed by any notice or attention that is given to him.

The period of adolescence is the last stage in the long process of growing up, the stage when the final weaning from emotional dependence on parents and the immediate family circle takes place. The young person turns outwards from the close emotional relationships with parents and home to form ties in the world outside. The ease with which this final break is accomplished depends on the satisfying nature of the relations with father, mother, brothers and sisters throughout childhood. If the young person's emotional needs at each stage of his development have not been satisfied he is not likely to feel secure enough to be ready to grow away from his home and to have sufficient confidence in his own emotional maturity to be able to build up warm and secure relations with other people. If he has never felt sure of his place in his family but retains feelings of jealousy he has been unable to resolve he is not likely to be able to free himself from feelings of rivalry and jealousy towards other young people and his capacity for forming normally friendly attachments will to that extent be diminished.

This final step towards independence is often greatly complicated for young people by the attitude of parents themselves. Some parents are not themselves mature enough to be able to accept this inevitable separation but unconsciously hold on to their children. In many different ways they meet their children's struggle towards independences with resistances of which they probably are not themselves aware.

Sometimes they do this by over-protecting their children, by standing between them and their world of reality. They insist on taking responsibility that the young person should long since have been encouraged to take for himself. They hold him back, whether they consciously mean to or not, from acquiring the skills necessary to act as a grown-up independent person.

Some parents also unconsciously hold on to their young people by playing on their feelings for them. Not long ago, a young nurse said to me: "I'm always unhappy when I've been home for a holiday because I feel so mean and selfish when I come away again. You see Daddy is away so much on business and Mummy is all alone except for me. She's so brave; she tries not to let me see how sad it makes her when I leave, but I can't help noticing it."

This situation is often made more difficult when there is only one parent. Geoffrey was seventeen. He had attempted to commit suicide and afterwards I saw him in hospital. His father had deserted his mother when Geoffrey was a few weeks old. Although she was left very poor she determined to do two things. She vowed first that she would never let Geoffrey really know what his father had done and second, that she would give

Geoffrey the kind of education that she would have chosen for him if his father had remained with them and her economic situation had been easier. In order to keep the first part of the vow she told Geoffrey, not that his father had gone away, but that he was dead. And to keep the second she undertook any work she could get, often of a very menial kind, to earn enough to send Geoffrey to a very good public school in London as a day boy.

When one talked to her it became clear that one of the factors in both these decisions was her own pride, although she always believed she was acting in Geoffrey's best interests. All through his school days Geoffrey and his mother lived in one furnished bed-sitting room. He could never invite friends home because his was not the kind of home which boys from that school were accustomed to visiting. He did well in his school-work and his mother provided for him in such a way that nobody at school suspected his poverty and the solitary life he led.

It is not to be wondered at, however, that as he grew up he became very restless and eager to break the emotional bonds with his mother and live a more normal lad's life. Wishing to do this he was filled with guilt at his own ingratitude toward this mother who, as she never hesitated to remind him, had sacrificed her whole life on his behalf because, as she expressed it, "he was all she had". The conflict became so great for him that he tried to resolve it in the only way that seemed possible to him—by committing suicide.

This boy of course had to meet with some very unusual and abnormal stresses. His mother, unhappy and rejected by her own husband, was seeking her own emotional satisfactions by trying to bind her son to her emotionally. Although this is a very extreme example the way in which many parents behave towards their children as they grow up is dictated by their own failure to achieve emotional maturity.

In our study of behaviour during later childhood we saw that boys and girls tended to go about in 'gangs' and to derive a certain amount of support from belonging to a group in which there was no great demand for intimacy of friendship. In adolescence the young person tends to withdraw from the gang and form deep and often very romantic friendships, at first with people of the same sex.

Later this kind of friendship is succeeded by friendship with someone of the opposite sex. Adolescence is the time when the young person experiments and gains experience in the emotions felt towards the opposite sex. These romantic, if immature, love affairs are the trial grounds out of which grow adult love leading to marriage and the foundation of a home and family.

One other problem which is very much to the forefront of the adolescent's mind is that of choosing a career and working to prepare for it. It is during this time that the young person needs not only the opportunity to learn to manage his own personal relationships with friends and colleagues but also to become aware of himself as a member of a community and to learn to accept the social responsibilities which that entails.

This final stage in the growing up process which takes place during adolescence thus involves:—

1. Physical growth from childhood to adulthood characterised chiefly by the maturing of the sex organs.

2. Intellectual growth towards a more abstract and mature mode of thinking.

3. The completion of the process of growth away from emotional dependence on parents in preparation for emotional relationships which will form the basis of adult relationships in marriage, in work and in the social community.

We have seen that this final growing-up period often puts considerable stress on the young person who is experiencing it. These stresses show themselves in the following characteristic ways:—

1. Alternation between childish and adult attitudes and modes of behaviour.

2. Marked variations in mood.

3. Variations between excessive bursts of energy and periods of laziness.

4. Retreat into solitariness, day-dreaming and phantasy.

5. Defiance of authority and behaviour that is argumentative and boastful: often as a cover for

6. Self-consciousness, awkwardness and feelings of inadequacy.

7. Extreme sensitiveness about the physical changes which are a part of adolescence.

Most student nurses are sufficiently close to their own adolescence to be able to understand much of this in the light of their own experience. If we examine what is happening to ourselves, what kinds of influences have affected us, why we feel and behave as we do towards different people, we can acquire understanding and tolerance of the patients under our care. If we can carry in our minds the kinds of problems that normally healthy adolescents are called on to face we can better appreciate that during a time of sickness in hospital they need all the tolerance and understanding that we can muster.

They need, above all, to be accepted as intelligent people who are capable of adult understanding, for nothing is so frustrating and irritating to an adolescent as to be talked down to as if he were a child. Some nurses adopt this manner of speech with all their patients. But whereas a fully mature adult may be able to tolerate it, even if with some amusement, the adolescent whose hold on 'grown-upness' is still so tenuous finds it very hard to bear.

It is important also to remember that a great many things that quickly become just a routine job for a nurse can be very embarrassing to an adolescent who is sensitive and self-consciously aware of his growing body. All the personal intimacies involved in the nursing care of a patient, carried out sometimes in a ward among patients of varying ages, can often seem to an adolescent a distressing encroachment on his personal privacy. An attitude which while matter of fact is at the same time not insensitive can be of very great help to adolescents in this respect.

These young people are often more worried and afraid than they like to show. It is a great help to them if the nurse explains as much as possible about the routine of the hospital and the procedure in relation to themselves, without waiting for them to ask. Very often indeed they would never be able to bring themselves to ask in case their questions should seem foolish.

Many adolescents are extremely reserved and we

should respect their reserve. While not trying to 'gate-crash' into their private world of thoughts and feelings, however, we should be readily interested in what they themselves want to tell us.

Although they often try by their behaviour to appear grown-up and independent, this façade frequently hides a great deal of insecurity and self-doubt, particularly during a time of illness. They need therefore, to feel that they are being cared for by people who have available for them consistently friendly support should they feel their need for it.

The patient who is the quietest and least demanding is not by any means always the most 'mentally healthy'. Many adolescents in times of great stress retreat from reality and try to find substitute satisfactions in a phantasy world of their own constructing. While this tendency to day-dreaming is common at some times in adolescence it is important to ensure that the young person in hospital is not too much forced in on himself by having nothing to do and nothing to interest him. It is now widely recognised that occupational interests contribute greatly to a patient's recovery. Nothing is so devastating to an adolescent as to have to lie aimless and idle while his roving mind is craving for interest and outlets. One very useful outlet is to give some measure of responsibility whenever it is possible. Young people are often greatly helped towards recovery by being allowed to participate responsibly in what is to be done for themselves or for others less able in the ward.

Before we leave this discussion of the adolescent let us look briefly at the kind of person he will have become when this final stage of his growth towards maturity is completed. He should be an individual personality in his own right, able to form his own judgments and make his own decisions regarding the rightness or wrongness of his actions. He should be capable of managing his personal relationships with other young people of either sex and with the adults with whom he now comes into contact in the widening sphere of his life. And he should be able to play his part responsibly as a member of the society to which he belongs.

CHAPTER IX

Adulthood

SO far in this book I have been describing the development of human behaviour throughout childhood and adolescence. I have given much more space to the study of the psychological aspects of this early period of growth than I shall to those of the adult period of life. In so doing I am following the plan rightly set out in the syllabus of the General Nursing Council, for the major pattern of the psychological growth of personality has been laid down by the end of adolescence and to understand the differing ways in which adults meet life and react to varying circumstances we need most of all to understand the basic necessities of sound personality growth in childhood and early youth. In the field of psychology it is very much the case that "the child is father of the man".

This natural pattern of development can of course be broken by accident or disease that damages the brain or the nerve cells or affects the proper functioning of certain glands. Brain damage occurring in an area which involves mental rather than physical functioning can alter not only intelligence but also feeling and behaviour. Marked changes in personality may be brought about by infections, such as, for example, some forms of encephalitis, meningitis or various forms of syphilis of the brain. There are also deteriorative conditions which usually occur in later life and may be due to haemorrhage or thrombosis in an area of the brain involving mental function. Sometimes this brings about changes in attitude and feeling in old people which it is difficult for relatives and friends to understand.

Sharp changes in mental functioning can also, of course, be brought about as a result of growths such as, for example, brain tumours while accidents involving head injuries may cause brain damage which results in sharp changes in the natural course of the development of behaviour.

I had a striking instance of this recently. Miss C. was brought into hospital with very severe head injuries caused by an accident when she was riding pillion on her fiancé's motor bicycle. She was just twenty-one when the accident occurred and she was to have been married the following week. It seemed at first unlikely that she could recover. She did, however, make a remarkable recovery. Physically the only damage was the loss of the sight of one eye. Even the scarring was minimal. Her personality, however, was completely changed. Before the accident she had been, according to descriptions given by her family and her supervisor and colleagues at work, gentle, reserved, sensitive and refined. She loved classical music and quiet, artistic pursuits. She was a telephonist and was regarded as a most responsible and reliable worker.

On recovery from the accident she was completely changed. She was noisy, vulgar and aggressive. She loved to pick a quarrel even with any stranger and would resort freely to loud, abusive language that filled those who were with her with embarrassment and shame. Although he felt guilty and distressed in doing it, her fiancé broke off the engagement because, as he put it, "it would be like marrying an entirely different person". Their interests which had formerly been very close were now quite dissimilar. For instance, one of their great pleasures had been going to the Promenade Concerts together but now she laughed such music to scorn and insisted that only jazz and be-bop were any good.

Miss C. attended the out-patients' department for some time after her discharge from hospital and it was during that time that I saw a good deal of her. She very quickly lost her job as a telephonist because she so easily resorted to vulgar abuse in her replies on the telephone or to her colleagues.

I examined her in hospital to see whether and in what ways her injuries had affected her mental functioning. Although she was so changed in attitudes and feeling her intellectual capacity was, in fact, impaired but little. It was difficult, however, to find an employer who could tolerate her for long because of her tempestuous, uninhibited behaviour. Her mother said to me, "I feel it's very wicked of me but I can't help wishing sometimes that she had never recovered because it's like having to get used to a completely different daughter. And she's too old now for me to bring her up in the way that I think right."

Nurses dealing with patients who have suffered from accidents or diseases such as I have described need to be aware of the fact that some accidents or diseases can alter personality and behaviour. But a more detailed discussion of the consequences of such illnesses is outside the scope of this book which is concerned with the development of the normal pattern of human behaviour in which, as I said earlier, what happens during childhood and adolescence is of major importance.

The ultimate goal in the development of a healthy personality is that of becoming an adult capable of acting on one's own initiative, of accepting responsibility for one's own actions, and of managing one's own personal relations with other people. To live satisfactorily in a community people must not only be integrated within themselves but also able to live in harmony with those who make up their world. It is only when one has become sufficiently adult to come to terms with one's own impulses and desires that one can do this and so reach what is the final stage in the progression to maturity—the ability to recognise and to accept emotionally the idea that the satisfactions, the happiness, and the security of other people is of equal importance to one's own.

Such recognition and acceptance is a necessary constituent of each of the main factors in adult living: participation in the social life of one's community, successful adjustment to the demands of whatever work one may be employed in, and the achievement of marriage and parenthood.

All life, however, is a changing and dynamic process. And just as there is no finality in physical health, so that adults for whom the time of physical growth and development is completed do not retain the same level of fitness and strength for the rest of their lives, so also there is no finality about mental and emotional health. Although the formative period of growth and development comes to an end with the end of adolescence, by which time the main patterns of our behaviour throughout life have been established, mental, physical and emotional change continues throughout the whole of life. Even those whose total development has been harmonious and satisfactory throughout these formative years can, under stress, lose for a time the steadiness of their emotional poise, while for those whose early emotional and mental development has been unsatisfactory the stresses of adult life can bring new crises. Each event in our lives influences the way in which our personality grows. The manner in which we meet each new experience is dictated by the pattern of our whole personality and by all that has happened to us previously. Moreover every phase of adult life brings its own particular problems and crises which make their own distinctive demand on our capacity to adjust.

Let us consider the main pattern of adjustment which each of these phases calls for; remembering always that it is even more true of the adult than the child—because the adult is, by the very fact of his maturity, at a more advanced and therefore more complicated level of personality than the child—that there is no such person as *the* adult, whether young, middle-aged or old, but that every individual varies. We can trace general principles which are common to all: we must be careful not to expect them to apply too rigorously in any one instance.

THE YOUNG ADULT.

The period of young adulthood can and should be one of the most exhilarating periods of life. The individual is now normally at the peak of his physical powers. If he is engaged on work that is vocationally 'right' for him he can find in it a satisfaction in the exercise of mature skill and the acceptance of adult responsibility such as the instabilities, self-doubts and emotional fluctuations inseparable from adolescence made impossible. It is a period also when the uncertainties which dog adolescent relationships are coming to an end and when the young adult is capable not only of forming more lasting ones with increasing confidence but also of accepting, without the anxieties which accompany the early stages of development, the demands of social intercourse at very many different levels of personal relationship.

Work, marriage, parenthood; these provide the major new experiences which in due course face the majority of young adults as they move forward from adolescence to full maturity. Each by its nature imposes strains and stresses that are to some extent different both in nature and degree from any of those met and dealt with earlier although the character of the response made by the individual to each of them will be conditioned by all that has gone to make up the pattern of his development from the very earliest stage of growth.

To adjust to the demands and responsibilities of a job is a practical necessity of life for the great majority of adults whether the nature of the occupation is the result of deliberate voluntary choice or has been dictated by circumstances. Where there has been deliberate choice the pleasure of accomplishing the first steps towards a desired ambition may be expected to ease the strain of adjustment to a new way of life with disciplines and obligations different from those earlier experienced. Yet such conditions may not always make for ease of adaptation to the new psychological situation which the beginning of work creates. The choice may have been on partial evidence, or on expectations with which the realities of the actual job conflict. As a result there may be a sense, if only temporarily, of frustration and disillusionment. Or else it may, for example, have been unconsciously dictated by identification with an admired figure—a father or mother—who has been successful in the same kind of work. In this way the sense of growing independence which is normally one of the most satisfactory accompaniments of the entry into adult employment may be overlaid and complicated by the emotional conflict resulting from the apparent inability to satisfy the psychological need to break free from the dependence of childhood. This was so in the case of the young nurse I mentioned in a previous chapter whose career was almost wrecked by her inability to adjust to the discipline and authority essential in a hospital although on the conscious level she was fully aware of their necessity and and was passionately anxious to fit in and make a success of her career. In this case it transpired that the girl's mother, whom she much admired but who had greatly dominated her in her youth, had before marriage had a very successful nursing career. The young nurse was torn between the urge to identify herself with her mother and the urge to become emotionally independent of her by challenging the authority she represented in the family relationship and had now—without the girl herself realising it—come to represent also in her life in the hospital.

Again the work chosen may, by the very fact that it has been attained as the result of a strong desire and a very positive ambition, set up anxieties as to one's ability to do all one had hoped—or all one's family circle has shown itself to expect. These anxieties may in themselves create tensions which make success more difficult.

Where the work has not been the result of deliberate choice but has been dictated by circumstances other tensions may well arise. The first job represents to a very significant degree the opening of the door upon adulthood for the adolescent or for the young man or woman. It is the first step towards economic independence and towards full acceptance as a grown-up person. But if it is uncongenial or boring or conflicts very markedly with the dreams and phantasies harboured, however unrealistically, during adolescence, then it may seem not so much to mark the opening of a door as the closing of one and to signify not, as it should, the gateway to the wider and more interesting country of adulthood but the final defeat of adolescent ambition.

Moreover although the beginning of working life brings with it a sense of independence it also imposes new disciplines which may well prove irksome, requiring as they do obedience to orders and the acceptance of a quite subordinate status in the new group. Such subordinate status may come particularly hard to those who have been very much the centre of interest and affection in their own homes or who have been people of importance in their community during their last years at school.

To these stresses are added in many industrial occupations the strain of repetitive work and of enforced concentration on tasks which may not in themselves hold the interest for long.

Such problems confront, in some degree or another, almost everyone. Most of us will be conscious of them in our experience and should be able to take account of them in dealing with other people. The adjustment to them is not too difficult for most reasonably well balanced people. It may, however, prove quite impossible for those whose early background has created serious emotional instability. The result is seen in a constant change of job, in an inability to settle down to any one type of occupation, and in lack of the power to mix happily with fellow workers or to accept the give and take of the office or workshop or the need to carry out orders without argument and resistance. But even amongst those who are, for the most part, well able to adjust to the new environment of their working life there may well be an onset of anxieties about their job in moments of tiredness or illness. Feelings of failure, jealousy of others thought to be more successful or believed to be preferred by those in authority, resentment of the obedience required by superiors or of the demands of a routine from which no escape seems possible: all these may at such times push themselves forward to attack our peace of mind.

The task of adjusting to the realities of the work-a-day life, of recognising and accepting the limitations imposed by circumstances, by one's own abilities or by economic factors which previously had little significance for us—all these are bound at times to bring with them tensions which may become particularly acute in periods of unhappiness or illness. For the normally stable person, however, none of them are likely to prove really serious.

The other major experiences that make big demands on the young adult's capacity for adjustment are those which centre round courtship and love leading to marriage and the making of a new home and later to the starting of a family.

Although love and courtship are in their first beginnings normally the result of physical attraction a mature relationship between two people of the opposite sex both demands, and also calls forth, a capacity for human association of the most adult kind. Such a relationship requires for its success the ability to regard another's well-being as no less or even more important than one's own and also the capacity to integrate one's personality with that of another. While it provides greater satisfactions than any other kind of human relationship it thus also makes greater demands. Moreover it does so, particularly in the early stages of courtship and marriage, when the heightened sensibilities which the emotion of love creates put even the most stable personality under an exceptional tension.

As in every other great crisis of emotional stress so, too, at this time patterns of behaviour belonging to earlier phases of development tend to be revived and repeated. In his need for an assurance and re-assurance of the unshakeable quality of his parents' regard for him an insecure child will, in early childhood, seek to secure it by testing out their love for him through behaviour which invites a rejection of him even though he dreads lest such a rejection should actually happen. Similarly during love and courtship the same urge to test out the steadfastness of the other person's affections—often in the most unreasonable ways is likely to arise, particularly for the person whose security is not firmly based. Nor is it surprising that at a time of such great emotional upheaval the feeling of jealousy which is common at an earlier phase of emotional development should easily be aroused.

Although such occasional jealousies are natural at times of intense emotion they are, however, unlikely to reach an uncontrollable level between people of a reasonably stable background. Courtship, culminating in marriage provides for most people one of the most happy and both emotionally and physically satisfying periods of their lives—a period during which the delicate and often complicated personal adjustments required on both sides are made possible and pleasurable by the excitement and happiness of mutual affection.

However deeply desired the arrival of the first child is bound to break into this intimate and delicately balanced relationship of man and wife. It is the first beginning of the change from a "you and I" pattern to a family pattern, with all its pleasures and happiness but also with all its needs for fresh adjustments. Starting a family initiates the acceptance of new and heavier responsibilities which in turn make greater demands on the maturity of the married couple.

Where the marriage is happy and satisfactory and the responsibilities are shared the personalities of both parents are likely to develop and be enriched by the mutual experience of loving and caring for their family. In such family care a happy, steadfast marriage between mature and stable people is the first essential. But even in the most mature relationship parenthood inevitably calls for great emotional adjustments.

In an earlier chapter I have described some of the continuing adjustments which the growing child is required to make in his feelings towards his parents and we have seen that it is normal for him to wish at times to separate them and play off one against the other. This growing-up process and the feelings which the child works through in his relation to his father and mother can very easily impose tensions on the other parties to it—the parents.

In the early weeks of a child's life there exists as we have seen earlier a bond between the infant and his mother which is by far the most important experience in the child's early years. During this time the part played by the father, while of great significance is nevertheless on the periphery, as it were, of the relationship between the mother and their child. His is the responsibility for making economic provision so that his wife can devote herself wholly to the care of their child and upon him also rests the duty of providing a background of emotional support and companionship which, by helping the mother to maintain a contented and untroubled mood, will create the peaceful and harmonious environment in which she and the child together can thrive.

The adjustments demanded of the young mother are dramatic and clearly determined. Those required of the father are less so and for this reason the extent to which the young father can, as it were, voluntarily relinquish for the time being his previous central position in his wife's thoughts and emotions and, stepping back, foster a relationship in which he at first seems to have only a minor part to play is an even greater measure of his adult stability.

Nor are the new adjustments called for by the ending of the "you and I" pattern which the arrival of the first child brings with it confined to the early days when it is perhaps easiest of all for the father to accept what may appear as a subordinate rôle, although actually one of the greatest importance. We have seen earlier that as a necessary part of the process of growing up a child has to accept the fact that there are other people in his environment; people who break in on that early one-to-one relationship which he has found so satisfying. The beginning of this acceptance comes through a relationship with the father. But young children cannot easily embrace two people in their loving at the same time and there are times, governed by the phase of development reached, when all children show intense feelings of jealousy towards one or other parent. In early childhood when the child's attachment to his mother is all-important to him there will, therefore, inevitably be many occasions when the father is forced to adjust himself to the fact that he is temporarily an object of jealousy and resentment to his children. Even the most mature may find this difficult to accept and tolerate unless they are able to appreciate its causes. Again in adolescence boys frequently pass through periods of great rivalry with their fathers and girls with their mothers.

Parents who are psychologically adult will find it possible to accept the fact that such emotions on the part of their children are natural and inevitable and will not themselves respond with anger and jealousy. Such an ability on the part of the parents to remain adult and not to regress in behaviour to the level of the child himself provides the security which is necessary to a child torn by the intensity of his own unstable emotions. It is not, however, always easy. In psychological work with parents and children who are emotionally sick one often meets parents who cannot make such adjustments; fathers, for example, who respond to their children's jealousies with the same emotion or mothers who foster this jealousy by playing off the son against the father.

In his account of research studies into the causes of family failure in Western communities Dr. Bowlby summarises the conclusions arrived at independently by psychologists and sociologists of high standing in two enquiries which were carried out in America in the 1930's. Although the two studies were quite independent of each other the following conclusions were common to them both. They agreed in finding that three factors were of major importance in married happiness:—

1. The marital happiness of the couple's parents.
2. The happiness of their childhood.
3. The affection of the husband and the wife for their own parents and particularly their good relationship with their own mothers.

From this they concluded that the love-life of the grown person is conditioned by his love relationships during childhood.

Because it continues to make heavy and changing demands on an adult's capacity for adjustment to new emotional situations parenthood is one of the great testing-grounds of an individual's maturity. Dr. Bowlby's report of research studies into the relationship between maternal care and mental health shows how difficult it is for deprived and unhappy children to grow up to make good parents. This is not surprising when we bear in mind that, as our own examination of the development of human behaviour has already made clear, the emotional maturity and stability of the adult has its roots in the satisfying quality of that person's childhood and adolescence within the family unit.

THE PERIOD OF MIDDLE AGE.

In this period of adult life emotional stresses and the needs for adjustment that arise out of them are naturally enough closely related to the physical changes that inevitably take place as the person grows older.

As the adult reaches middle age, usually in the forties, he becomes aware of physiological changes which point to the beginning of a decline in physical capacity even though slow at first. We all know that in some sports the athlete has reached the peak of his powers as early as the middle twenties. For a time he may make up for the decline in fine physical skills by his increased maturity of judgment and wisdom but gradually his declining physical ability makes it necessary for him to retire. Of course the change for average people is neither so early nor so sharply marked as for the professional sportsman and they can continue to enjoy their game of tennis or golf while making a gradual adjustment to their slowly declining physical powers.

In the intellectual field although the actual growth of intellectual capacity probably comes to an end in early maturity, new learning, new ideas, new experiences combine to provide a maturity of judgment that remains effective much longer than the lessons of experience can for the athlete. Studies of adult intelligence go to show, however, that some aspects of intellectual ability decline more markedly than others. Throughout middle age people find, for example, that they become less quick in assimilating new ideas and cannot so readily retain and recall what they learn. These changes present constant problems of adjustment for the person who is growing older.

Just as for girls the beginning of menstruation demands a sharper adjustment to growing up and to sexual maturing than in the case of boys, so in her middle years the woman is faced more sharply than is a man with the need to accept the fact of ageing. With the onset of the menopause a woman must accept the physical fact of the cessation of her capacity for child-bearing. Quite often for the married woman the physical changes caused by the menopause and the inevitable sense of loss that goes with it coincides with the growing up of the family when children are increasingly less dependent on their home and parents for interests and satisfactions. This comes as a sharp reminder to the mother that the pattern of her life, according to which her main activity and interest has centred on her family's need of her, is changing. Her success in adjusting to these changes will be determined by the extent to which she has been able to recognise the need to prepare herself gradually to meet them. It will be easiest if she has not allowed her children to absorb her wholly but has continued to foster her friendship with her husband and retain and also extend her interests in the world outside her home.

For the childless woman the menopause marks the end of any hope of bearing children of her own, and for the single woman it represents a lessening of the possibility of marriage.

The changes brought by middle age are much less sharp for men. Men are also helped by the fact that their work, which for most people provides one of their main interests, does not end when their children grow up and leave home. The process of growing older, therefore, is not so critically dramatic for men as it is for women and particularly for married women whose main career has circled round the care and upbringing of their children. Mothers who are not sufficiently well adjusted within themselves to be able to see in these changes opportunities to widen their own horizons and enrich their experience often make the business of growing towards independence a very difficult one for their children. A mother who has not developed interests that can continue apart from her life with her children will inevitably be impelled to seek satisfactions from their lives and will thus hold on to them, at any rate emotionally, long after they should have been free to grow up and away from her.

Those parents whose own lives have not been emotionally satisfying tend to feel jealous of their own children as they grow up, particularly if their lives are full and happy. Often in my work as a psychologist I have to listen to complaints by parents of their adolescent sons and daughters and the problems and difficulties which they present. Very frequently, however, it seems more true that the real difficulties lie in the fact that the parents themselves are failing to adjust to a changing situation in their own lives. For it is an essential part of maturity to be able to embrace each new phase of life as it comes and to welcome each new experience even if it brings with it big demands for emotional adjustment. Only in this way can people avoid looking back upon their lives with a sense of dissatisfaction and regret for what they have missed.

THE PERIOD OF OLD AGE.

The fact of ageing is in itself a very difficult reality for most people to face and accept. It compels adjustments in every person's way of life of which the major ones centre round three main causes:— those demanded by the need to recognise and accept the fact that both physical strength and also intellectual ability are declining, those called for by the new pattern of living which comes with retirement from one's job, and the emotional adjustments which change of status within the family group and the progressively increasing loneliness and bereavements which are the inevitable concomitants of age all call for.

Every human capacity, after attaining a maximum, begins to decline. This decline is progressive but it is at first so slow as to be almost imperceptible. Throughout the period of early adult life and well on into middle age most healthy people are not unduly conscious of the slow decline in their mental or physical capacities. The most noticeable decline is in the sensory field. Vision and hearing fall off rapidly after the age of about 30. In the sixties, however, the reality of ageing becomes much more obtrusive because of an all-round, general decline in physical capacity. Men and women of this age become more sharply aware of the limits of their energy and vital capacity because they reach these limits so much more quickly with so much less achievement than when they were at the height of their physical and mental powers. Many become acutely conscious, also, of not seeing so well and not hearing so well. This general limiting of ability creates for elderly people a feeling of isolation. This is particularly so when loss of hearing is severe.

A considerable body of research into adult intelligence and deterioration with age goes to suggest that intellectual abilities also show a slow but progressive impairment with age. Dr. David Wechsler, Chief Psychologist at the Bellevue Psychiatric Hospital, New York, who has made a vast contribution to knowledge in this field by his research studies of adult intelligence and modes of assessing it, found that, apart from decline in sensory acuity, particularly in sight and hearing, many of our mental abilities show greater impairment with age than do our physical ones. But, as I pointed out earlier, what a person loses through the gradual falling off of innate ability is, throughout most of adult life, made up for by greater acquired knowledge and wider experience. Thus to quote Wechsler, "an old clinician may be a better doctor than a younger one, even though he possesses less actual understanding of disease processes".

The big change which we associate with old age comes when the all-round decline in capacity begins to impose severe limitations on the ability to reach out for new experiences of body and mind and for that new knowledge on which both mind and body feed.

Throughout life our adjustment to each new phase in our development is made within a framework of physical and intellectual capacity which is inherent. The more readily the limitations of this inherent capacity are recognised, the more smoothly will the adjustments called for by each new phase be made. With the approach of old age, however, this inherent capacity itself declines noticeably and adjustments have to be made within a framework which is itself becoming more limiting.

The big adjustment required of the individual who is entering upon the period of old age is, therefore, to accept the fact that because every organism suffers an all-round decline with the process of senescence this will inevitably, even though gradually, impose limitations on what one can do both in a physical and intellectual sphere. Having recognised this as an immutable condition within which to plan the person who is stable and mature can find ways of living which continue to provide new and rewarding satisfactions through the period of old age.

Some people, and particularly those who feel that their earlier life has not provided all the satisfactions it should have done, cannot however easily adjust to the fact that age does impose these immutable limitations. According to temperament they either defy it unreasonably or else accept it so fatalistically that they 'give in' more than is necessary. The former refuse to recognise warning signs that their physical strength and powers are not as great as they were. They consistently overtax their strength with the result, very often, that they risk a physical disaster which may well force upon them a much greater adjustment to permanent incapacity. The latter tend to abandon even such activities as would be perfectly possible. 'Because they are old now' they feel they cannot get out as they used to, they cannot bother to see people, they cannot do this or that and they sit back and allow the ageing process to close in on them and limit their lives so that the deterioration associated with senescence is in this way speeded up.

The examination of the brains of patients who suffered from senile dementia prior to death frequently reveals what are described as senile plaques on the cerebral cortex. Research has shown however that there is no relationship between the incidence of such structural changes in the brain and impairment of mental function. It has in fact been proved that mental deterioration is very slight indeed in those intellectual functions that are practised and used in the life of the ageing individual and that old people in institutions become senile and helpless much more quickly if they are kept in bed with nothing to do and with no interests. They are healthiest, both mentally and physically, if they are encouraged to get up and take some responsibility for and interest in a real job of some sort however simple. Within the limitations of the slow process of decline in capacity, therefore, the mature and well-balanced person will find interests and satisfying ways in which to use his time; he will keep his mind alive to new ideas and reach out, as far as it is possible, to meet new experiences.

For many people the sharpest adjustment to the fact of ageing come with retirement. This is particularly so because at the same time as it sharply deprives the person of the occupations and interests that have absorbed most of his waking hours, retirement also brings with it the need for a difficult emotional readjustment. For most people it represents, or appears to represent, a loss of status that they find difficult to accept. And in any case it necessitates a readjustment in habits and way of life that often affects the whole household.

As an illustration of the difference in the level of maturity shown in the capacity to accept retirement two men come into my mind. Both these men reached retiring age at about the same time so that for me the contrast was more vividly marked.

One was the Managing Director of a Company who for at least two years before retiring allowed himself to become progressively more embittered as the time for his retirement inevitably drew nearer. He could not tolerate the loss of status and feeling of importance that his position had given him. Since retiring he has devoted a large proportion of his time to making his successor's life difficult by his interference. Almost daily he sends long reams of written instructions and criticism of the way in which the younger man is filling "his" post.

The other, a man of great brilliance in the field of

science, prepared with considerable wisdom and forthought for the time of his retirement. He gradually built up for himself an ever-widening sphere of interests and accepted positions on a variety of committees and public services of a kind which were useful and valuable to the community but which could only be undertaken by people with leisure.

Throughout his life he had been physically a very active person and was a very keen mountaineer. As climbing became gradually less possible for him, he found other leisure time pursuits which would give him lively interests and take him out of doors among the kind of scenery that he loved. He took up painting with all the verve and enthusiasm of a much younger person. To him the period of retirement became a time to widen his range of experience and interest in ways that had been impossible during a tightly packed working life. As a consequence of this he is still active, vigorous and alert of mind and a most interesting and lively person to be with. He has, as he himself expresses it "come to terms with old age". By accepting the limits which his age imposes on him he has made it possible to live life very fully within them.

The other man has allowed his interests to become narrowed and has closed himself off from the world. He rarely goes out or meets other people. He is always disgruntled and hostile in his attitude to any new idea expressed by a younger person. He suffers from an increasing number of aches and pains and physical disabilities and is rapidly becoming an old man in the full meaning of the term.

The adjustment to retirement demands real maturity on the part of the ageing person. It is not easy to accept the fact that the time has rightly come to stand aside and allow younger people to take more responsible jobs while one undertakes work which seems of much less importance. Many people continue to hold on to their job, creating frustration and despair for the younger people who are ready to accept more responsibility.

This is likely to become more of a problem in a society such as ours whose population is because of increased medical skills and better provisions for health and hygiene an ageing one.

Though it must be met in part by the planning and forethought of the stable and well-balanced individual himself, elderly people can also be helped quite considerably by adjustments which take proper account of the problem.

Some of the more enlightened local authorities now organise part-time employment schemes for old people who are enabled to carry out simple tasks in short working shifts. They are usually paid a small flat-rate and as the work some of them can do is often not very profitable, such schemes often cost more to run than the old people can actually earn. But by taking these old people out of their homes—and incidentally giving some relief to those who care for them—by giving them the sense of having something worth while to do, and by enriching their lives with new experiences and friendships with their own contemporaries, senility is kept at bay and the real saving is thus immeasurable. A similar end is served by social clubs for old people.

Old people are happiest and best cared for within their own family community and not in institutions and hospitals. With an ageing community and smaller families and homes this is not always so easy as it was in Victorian days. Provision for old people is therefore tending to be accepted as a shared responsibility of the community. Schemes for part-time work, social clubs and cottage homes with some home help and also nursing care available, offer the best solution. In this way old people can remain in their own family community without this placing too great a burden of care for them on the younger generations growing up who, at the same time, continue to accept some responsibility for their ageing parents.

During a visit to the mental hospitals of one State in the U.S.A. I learnt that 50 per cent of the patients in the State Mental Hospitals were old people who were not mental patients at all in the real sense of the term. Their only reason for being there was that they were old and that the urban conditions and way of life in modern American cities made it impossible for their families to care for them at home.

This is not only wasteful of nursing facilities—and these hospitals were grossly overcrowded in consequence—but it is also a denial of the real human needs of the aged and a thwarting of the true pattern of the family community. To this pattern old age, no less than youth and middle age, has much to contribute and in it the natural affection and respect of youth for age should have a valuable part.

Perhaps one of the most difficult of all the adjustments of old age is the emotional adjustment to the change in status within the family and to increasing loneliness. It is inevitable that people who grow to old age lose many of their contemporares and find themselves more and more as time passes in a world of younger people with different interests and a different background of memories and associations. Those whose job involves the care of old people need to appreciate the intensity of loneliness that old people can suffer as one by one their contemporaries, their friends and their relations die. This often arouses in some of them very real fears and worries as to what will happen to them as they become more and more childlike in their dependence on other people and in their need for the sense of security that this can give. But although in their dependence and need for care old people may seem to be like children, the saying "Once a man and twice a child" is very misleading. The old are not children but men and women who, although their capacities are now in the natural order of things declining have behind them great richness of experience and service, To treat them as children is humiliating and unkind. It is to ignore all that lies behind them and in so doing to affront the dignity and respect that age should carry with it.

It is important to remember that old people vary greatly in their sensitivity regarding their dependence on other people for the personal care that they can no longer undertake for themselves. They differ also in the extent to which they can, without anxiety, accept their increasing loneliness and face the reality of death. Most old people seek solace for this loneliness by living more and more in the past. Aged people love to recount stories of their childhood and to recall such memories over and over again, often to the exasperation and boredom of younger people who have to listen to them. But if we bear in mind the kind of difficulties and anxieties that beset old people and the stresses they have to meet, their behaviour, even when because of those stresses it is trying or incalculable, becomes easier to understand and therefore to tolerate.

CHAPTER X

Human Behaviour in Health and Sickness

WHEN we speak of human behaviour, we mean the way in which human beings react to their immediate circumstances, not only what they do but also what they say, the way they look, the expressions of emotion that they show. All that we know about other people originates from our own experience; every new event in our own lives is experienced in the light of what has happened earlier. No new experience, therefore, is met completely without bias: it is always coloured by the interests and attitudes that have grown out of our earlier experiences. Moreover not only is our experience always changing but the impact of each new experience also changes us. No event is ever, therefore, seen or experienced in exactly the same way by two different people for nothing that happens is identically the same for any two people. Moreover, we never become actively aware of or perceive all the stimuli that impinge on our senses. This is because our selection of the things that we see and the events that we take notice of in our lives, as well as the things that we ignore and allow to pass us by, is dictated by attitudes and interests that have grown out of our previous experiences. It follows that no two people behave exactly alike because even if they are exposed to the same event they do not bring the same experience to bear on it. And because it has a different meaning for them they react to it in different ways.

"Two men looked through prison bars;
One saw mud, the other stars."

Those whose job involves working with and understanding people need to recognise the complexity of human behaviour. It is never simple nor influenced by motives that are single and clear-cut. It is always dynamic and changing. And reactions to events are always different for different people.

One of the basic needs of all human beings is to feel secure in their social relationships. The extent to which they feel confident in their dealings with other people depends mainly on their feelings about themselves. We saw earlier that an emotionally disturbed child is one who has lost his assurance that he is regarded as a worthwhile person by the people who are important in his life and whom he loves and needs. Similarly a grown-up's attitude to other people and his capacity for forming satisfying human relationships derives from his perception of himself and from his idea of what other people think of him—whether he feels himself to be liked and wanted, or disliked and unwanted, inferior, equal or superior to other people in his community.

In our study of the development of behaviour we have seen that an individual can only achieve the full maturing of his personality and character through human relationships. Human beings cannot live in isolation and for most people the greatest unhappiness and fear is aroused by the feeling of being disapproved of and rejected by the people who make up their world. It is from the incentive which this essential need to be approved of and accepted provides that people develop the ability to control their immediate impulses and repress those of their wishes and desires which meet with social disapproval.

Nobody can easily give up his own wishes entirely and there is always a certain conflict in the individual between his desire to satisfy his own impulses and his need to be accepted by other people in his community. Anxiety is aroused for most people when the security of their good relationship with, and the assurance of their own worth whileness in relation to the people who make up their community is challenged. The kind of situations which arouse this anxiety and the ways in which people deal with it differ from person to person. Much of human behaviour is influenced by the need to protect this urge for security in social relationships or to restore it when it has been shaken or lost. And it is in the light of this that all human behaviour has a significance and a meaning.

We cannot ever wholly judge the meaning that any experience has for another person because we can only see it in terms of our own experience. Moreover we cannot ever entirely know a person as he is within himself and we are largely influenced in our judgment of him by the impact which his behaviour makes on us personally. Before we can properly begin to understand other people we need, therefore, to recognise that what we notice about other people and how we feel about them is determined largely within ourselves, by our own past experiences, our interests and attitudes and that in order to have some psychological insight into the behaviour of others we must understand the part that we ourselves are playing in the relationship which has developed between us. At the same time it is necessary to make a deliberate effort of the imagination to seek to understand another's point of view, to "put ourselves in their place" as the common saying has it.

It is only when we can recognise and accept these facts

that we can begin to observe human behaviour more objectively.

Yet even although it is necessary always to bear in mind that no two human beings are exactly alike and no single event has the same significance for any two individuals there are certain characteristic patterns of behaviour which are commonly adopted by most people and which it is therefore helpful for those who are in their work concerned with the well-being of other people to be able to recognise and understand.

These attitudes or ways of thinking, or, to use the psychological term, these *mental mechanisms*, are adopted in order to resolve or at least keep in check the anxiety that arises when a person's security regarding his social relationships and consequently his confidence in his own worthwhileness is shaken. They are never completely uncomplicated, nor are they thought out and adopted with any conscious purpose. To describe them separately, as we must, inevitably makes them seem much simpler and more clear-cut than they really are. In actual behaviour they overlap and become confused with many other factors and it is often impossible to identify them exclusively.

Perhaps one of the most obvious ways of trying to defeat anxiety if only temporarily—one which we probably have all used at some time to some extent—is to deny that any reason for the anxiety exists. This of course never leads to a satisfactory solution nor does it achieve its goal of defeating anxiety.

The parents of Roger, a seven-year old boy came to me for advice because their son was so backward in school. They had entered him for one of the more academic of our public schools and they were worried that he would not be able to pass the entrance examination for its preparatory school. On tests the boy proved to be very dull indeed, on the borders of mental defect, and he had not learnt to read or do numbers because such tasks were quite beyond the level of his intellectual capacity at that time. When I tried to explain this to the parents and to point out to them that the kind of ambitions they had for their son could not possibly be realised they were angry with me and insisted that I was wrong.

Roger is now nine years old and his parents have taken him from school to school and hospital to hospital in the hope of finding somebody who will tell them what they themselves wish to believe—that he is a clever boy whose failure to learn is due to laziness. By now, as is only to be expected, Roger is a very anxious, maladjusted child. He is not only failing to learn but he also wets and soils, steals and truants. But his parents are still seeking to reduce the severity of their very great anxiety by denying that there are any real grounds for it. This is, of course, a very extreme case for the parents are themselves deeply neurotic people but it serves as a more than usually clear-cut example of an attempt to reduce anxiety by adopting a single mode of thought and denying all evidence that their view is wrong.

There is a tendency in all human beings to explain events—and this applies particularly to unhappy events—in personal terms. In work with children who are born with severe physical handicaps, such as deafness or blindness or paralysis, or with children with mental defect one often finds that the parents bear within themselves a deep sense of guilt. It is as though, albeit without realising it, they blame themselves and their own inadequacy for the handicaps under which their children suffer. In the case of Roger it is reasonable to suppose that the child's failure deeply challenged the parents' sense of their own adequacy as people and that the motives which impelled them to behave as they did were much more complex than the single reason which they constantly expressed—namely that they were determined to give their son the best education and preparation for adult life that money could buy.

Repression is a more complicated mechanism by which emotions that are too unpleasant for a person to accept are pushed out of consciousness and forgotten. We can all probably recall occasions in our lives when we have deliberately pushed out of our minds some thought or emotion that was either unpleasant or with which it was not appropriate at that particular time to deal. Repression, however, is quite different from such a conscious act of control. We owe our concept of it to Freud. It was part of Freud's thesis that many of the turbulent feelings of early childhood, feelings which though highly charged with emotion it was socially unacceptable to express and therefore frightening to recognise, were so deeply repressed as to be virtually completely forgotten and in this way the child's self-regard particularly in relation to his parents was protected. Freud held that this repressed material was frequently so strongly charged with emotion that it could continue powerfully to influence behaviour without the individual being aware of it. It was no small part of his contribution to psychopathology that he found ways of bringing back to consciousness, and thus resolving, the conflict that had gathered round such of the repressed material as was a source of mental ill-health to his patients.

Explanations of the ways by which repressed feelings and emotions motivate a person's behaviour are still in the area of controversy and a vast field for research lies ahead. Many of the theories postulated by Freud and his successors have yet to undergo that long process of experimental testing and trial from which a body of verifiable information can be built up in the way in which all scientific knowledge is extended. Nevertheless the truth of many of the theoretical hypotheses put forward by Freud and others has been empirically demonstrated in the successful treatment of the mentally sick. It is not unreasonable to suggest that for many sick people coming into hospital as patients and having to accept the dependence on others that being in hospital necessarily imposes attitudes and feelings related to the period of their childhood when they were normally dependent on other people are also revived. For those people who have never adequately resolved the conflicts associated with this period, behaviour in hospital towards those on whom they now depend is coloured by the feelings they had towards their parents in early childhood. It can then happen that their behaviour towards the nurse or the doctor is influenced without their realising it by repressed emotions which do not relate to anything in the personality or behaviour of the nurse or doctor but have become attached to them as authoritative figures in this new condition of dependence in which the patients find themselves.

Projection is a very usual method of resolving conflicts and safeguarding one's self-esteem. Like most mental mechanisms it does not take place consciously. Projection is the act of attributing feelings, thoughts or activities which in reality have their origin within our own personality, to any individual other than ourselves. Some examples may make this clearer. Projection occurs when we interpret the feelings or actions of another person in terms of our own feelings and wishes. We harbour feelings of hostility and hatred towards a person but those are feelings to which it would be damaging to our self-esteem to admit. So instead of saying "I hate her and would like to destroy her", we say and genuinely believe, "She hates me and I think she would like to destroy me".

Projection is resorted to, also, when we attribute to other people those faults of which we are most aware but often cannot acknowledge within ourselves. A head-mistress of my acquaintance complained of every student teacher under her supervision, that she could not control her class and keep order. It was some time before I learnt by chance that her own career as a teacher had nearly come to an untimely end because she herself had had the greatest trouble in keeping order in her classes. As soon as she was in a position of authority she bolstered up her own self-regard by attributing to others her own personal failing. We all tend to resort to projection at times without our being aware of it. We all assume that we know by the things he says what another person thinks or feels and what are the motives that lie behind his actions but we only really know what we can infer from our own similar words and actions regarding the experiences which lie behind them.

An awareness of the general human tendency to project, is of inestimable aid in a job such as nursing where so much turns on the ability to manage human relationships and where the nature of the work involves a much more constant and intimate association with colleagues than is the case with a daily job in an office or factory. For example a nurse who is convinced that the ward sister dislikes her may find if she can look deep enough that in truth she herself is projecting on to the sister her own inner feelings of dislike.

These then are but a few of the mental mechanisms that people frequently adopt to protect their self-regard and in that way to defeat the anxiety that arises from feelings of conflict and insecurity in their human relationships within their community. Human emotions are very complex and the methods which people adopt to deal with them in order to retain both their own personal integration and their harmonious relations with the world outside are not only both varied and complicated but usually lie outside the conscious awareness of the individual himself.

During the whole of life an unceasing demand is made on all individuals for adjustment to changing situations. The healthy person can meet these demands without undue stress. But it is none the less true of adults as we saw it to be in the case of children that physical illness places an added strain on people. By it increased demands are made on their capacity to adjust.

Throughout this book I have sought to emphasise the closeness of the interaction between an individual's mind, body and emotions and to stress the truth that a person's thoughts and his feelings contribute quite as much as does his physical condition to both health and ill-health. Just as an individual's physical health affects his thoughts and feelings so also his physical health is greatly affected by them.

It is many years since a famous French physician said that there are no diseases, but only sick people. It is important always to bear this in mind. In order to make it easier to recognise, as it were, the sick person behind the disease, I will describe briefly some of the more characteristic ways in which people react to physical illness. These reactions vary greatly in different individuals but they are all, in their separate ways, expressions of the anxiety that being ill has aroused in them and they can best be understood in the light of every human being's basic need to be accepted by his community and to feel secure in his relationships with the people who form his world.

Human behaviour in illness, therefore, varies according to the temperament, the past experience, and the significance that being ill has for the individual who is experiencing it. For most people it diminishes their sense of total well-being and consequently lowers their self-regard. Behaviour is directed towards restoring this self-regard or at any rate protecting or readjusting to what remains of it. Because, as we saw earlier, people tend to explain unhappy events in personal terms, being ill arouses in many people a deep sense of guilt. They feel, without being consciously aware of it, that they are being punished for some failure within themselves.

For some people this feeling of their own inadequacy is so great that they protect themselves from any new risk of failing in human relationships by withdrawing from association with other people. They become apathetic and depressed and try to close themselves off from their surroundings and from associating with other people. This unfortunately increases their loneliness and feeling of rejection.

Others, however, seek to restore their belief in themselves by blaming, not themselves but other people or circumstances for the misfortune that has befallen them. These people are critical, complaining, and frequently openly hostile. This kind of behaviour is unfortunate where it occurs among people who cannot understand its significance and consequently make some allowance for it. It is a sick person's way of trying to restore his belief in himself particularly with regard to his relationships with other people and if it is met by hostility and aggression it confirms that person's doubts and defeats its own purpose.

Some people concentrate almost entirely on the physical aspect of their disease. It is a characteristic pattern of the behaviour of certain people to use physical illness as, one might almost say, a weapon with which to secure the attention of others. They complain of many aches and pains and physical discomforts for which no organic cause can be found. Such physical ailments serve to reduce the demands that are made on them and also win for them a certain amount of extra sympathy and attention.

It is important however not to minimise the effect of emotion and particularly the emotions of fear and anxiety on physical well-being. Strong emotions always have a physical accompaniment.

It is not necessary to think of times of illness in order to recall events which, because they have aroused emotional tensions of some kind or another, have also been accompanied by bodily reactions. Some people always have diarrhoea or are sick before an examination, some tremble when they are afraid and such phrases as "he was so alarmed that he broke out into a cold sweat" or "his heart beat rapidly for joy" or "he was too excited to sleep" are common to our language.

Although, to take one example, it has been long recognised that strong emotion affects digestion, it has in more recent times been scientifically demonstrated by exact and carefully planned observations how closely what a person thinks or feels, that is, the meaning that every event has for him, is reflected by physical changes in the stomach.

Anxiety and tension lasting over a long period, therefore, are closely associated with serious digestive disorders such as gastric ulceration. Certain illnesses, such as gastric or duodenal ulcers, many skin diseases, some forms of rheumatism and asthma, some forms of blood pressure and some heart diseases have been described as "psycho-somatic" illnesses, because psychological factors are so closely involved both in their onset and treatment.

It is not surprising, therefore, that the great emotional stresses which being physically ill inevitably create for most people affect the condition and functioning of the body in a wide variety of ways.

It is a characteristic reaction of nearly all human beings under stress and difficulty to regress to a more childish level of behaviour. It is a way, although often to others it does not seem to be a very sensible or even successful way, of seeking security and reassurance. It is not surprising, therefore, to meet in hospital even among adult patients, those who are unreasonably demanding or fretful and querulous, those who are watchful for what seems to them unfair treatment, those who are excessively dependent, those who are outspokenly afraid or those who deliberately set themselves to annoy and irritate other patients; all these are among the many forms of immature and childish behaviour to which anxious, disturbed or unhappy people frequently resort.

Whatever form a sick person's behaviour takes, it is his expression of the meaning that his experience has for him; it is his characteristic and unique way of reacting to that particular environment and by his behaviour he is expressing something more about himself than can be conveyed in words.

CHAPTER XI

The Sick Patient in Hospital

IT now remains to apply what we have learnt from this study of the psychology of human nature, its development, its variations and its needs, to the care of sick people in hospital.

We have already seen that all human beings are required constantly to adjust themselves to changing experiences and that they do this in the course of healthy, normal living. But although normal demands for adjustment are being made of people throughout the whole of life there are also times when the stresses caused by changes of experience are so great that the capacity of the individual to adjust to them is stretched to the uttermost. This increased tension shows itself in an infinite variety of ways according to the inherited characteristics and also the past experiences of the individual undergoing them.

The experience of physical illness or disease together with its effect on the mind and feelings of the sick person brings with it changes that create their own demands for adjustment. In any dealings with sick people under whatever circumstances it is important that due recognition should be given to this.

But our particular concern in this chapter is with the extra difficulties and tensions that are created for a person who is a patient in hospital and the ways in which the pressure of anxiety which they create can be reduced by the understanding and particularly by the psychological insight of the nurse.

It is convenient to think of the time spent by a patient in hospital as falling into three phases: the initial period of his entry into hospital when he is being settled in in preparation for whatever treatment he is to undergo, the period of treatment proper, and the period of convalescence when he is preparing to take up normal living again. Each of these periods presents its own peculiar demands on the individual's capacity to adjust to it.

Coming into hospital as a sick patient constitutes for most people a very sharp and extensive change of experience. First, and perhaps most traumatic of all, it brings about a complete severance from the human or social environment to which the patient normally belongs. It separates him, for the time being at any rate, from his family, his work or his school, his leisure interests—from everything, in fact, that constitutes the community to which he 'belongs' and through his relationships to which he has built up his own self-esteem. Man is a social being and his deep-seated need for security in social relationships influences his behaviour at every point of his life. The temporary uprooting from his settled social pattern caused by coming into hospital shakes this security in his relation to people at a time when his own feeling of "disease" has inevitably diminished his belief in his own adequacy and worth. Here then he is faced with forming a new pattern of relationships with people who are complete strangers to him and towards whom he is in a particularly dependent position.

This adjustment is made more difficult by the fact that coming into hospital as a patient involves a complete change in a person's physical environment and a break from all the familiar things of home which give a sense of continuity in his life. For many people the strangeness and the large, institution-like character of the building, the unfamiliar bed in a ward full of people whom one does not know, the difference in food, meal-times, times of waking and times of settling for sleep, the whole change in routine—all these things add, in varying degrees depending on the temperament and inner stability of the person experiencing them, to the fear and alarm which this new and strange situation arouses. Many people also find it very difficult to accept what seems to them a violation of their personal privacy such as takes place for example when they are washed or use the bed-pan, although for the nurse such things have long since become part of the every day routine of her work. How difficult adjustment to the new set of circumstances demanded by the entry into hospital and the early 'settling in' period proves will depend most of all on the inner emotional adjustment and basic security of the individual concerned. Much also depends, of course, on the severity of the illness that has brought the patient to hospital. A very sick person may experience only relief that at last he has come under the care of experienced doctors and nurses who can take entire responsibility for him until he is restored to health again.

For most people, however, the initial experience of leaving home and coming into hospital and the early period of settling in with all the adjustments it involves, when added to the very real fears aroused by the illness itself, creates an anxiety which it is the part of the job of the hospital staff to recognise and help to alleviate. There are many ways in which the nurse can contribute to doing this.

The difficulty of adjusting to new surroundings and a new set of circumstances can be greatly lessened for a patient by straightforward explanations of hospital conditions and procedure and details of ward routine—all the information indeed, however simple and obvious it may have come to seem to the nurse, that it is useful or necessary for a patient to have. It is helpful also to try to anticipate and answer those questions which many patients may be too shy or self-conscious to ask for themselves.

Patients often express fears for which the nurse may know there are no real grounds. As in the case of children we can best help them to overcome these fears if we recognise that for them they are very real. We have already seen that by trying to 'jockey' a child out of his fear by laughing at him and insisting that there is nothing to be afraid of, as we ourselves may genuinely believe, we are in fact placing a barrier between ourselves and the child which makes it difficult for us to help him. We present ourselves as someone who cannot understand how real this fear is though the reality of it still remains with the child.

So also in dealing with sick adults we can, even when their fears seem to us quite unreasoned, help them best if, while trying by explanations to show them that their fears are groundless, we also show that we recognise that they are very real to them and for that reason we take them seriously. Many of these fears in fact disappear when necessary explanations are given at a level at which people can understand and when they feel they are being told the truth.

It is in all these ways that a nurse shows her good feeling for her patients. During their time in hospital it is the nurse who comes into closest and most continuous contact with them so that in this new situation in which the patient is of necessity adjusting to a new pattern of social relationships a realisation of the good feeling that the nurse has for him is of paramount importance to his well-being. In order to foster this good feeling it is necessary to recognise that each individual patient is a unique personality who reacts to illness with his body, mind and emotions in his own individual way. It follows that one must remember always that one is not called upon to nurse an appendix or a septic throat or whatever the physical illness may be, but a sick person. When that is recognised it is easier to accept more objectively the vagaries of behaviour that the experience of being in hospital calls out in different people, and as a result to preserve one's good feeling towards them all. We cannot do this if we pigeon-hole people in our minds in terms of the nature of their illness, their age, their sex or any other mode of grouping them. And although it is of value to have a clear mental picture of the reasons for, and the characteristics of behaviour at all the various developmental levels from birth to maturity, it is equally important to remember always the uniqueness of every individual.

The other day in a hospital ward an elderly woman showed great anxiety to speak to me privately. She was Miss X, a 78 years old maiden lady who had a badly fractured femur as a result of a fall. She looked fretful and unhappy. I went over to her to see what she wanted and she drew me to her and whispered, "Will you tell the nurses that I'm *not* a granny. They keep calling me 'Granny' even though I've told them I'm not a granny. I was never married you know." As I talked to her it became clear that she was a person who had always wanted to marry and felt her failure to marry and have children very deeply. Being called Granny when she was old and ill was bringing back emotions of frustration and sorrow that could not help but impede her recovery.

As I went out, I told the nurse what she had said. She laughed brightly and replied, "Oh, but we call all the old dears Granny".

For that particular nurse all the old people who came under her care were grouped together in her mind as "old dears". I have no doubt that, according to the limits of her understanding, she gave them good care and nursing, But she could never really give them the best nursing care until she could learn to see them all as individual people —all alike in being old, but all very different in their experiences and backgrounds, in their feelings and fears and likes and dislikes.

This kind of good feeling which has its roots in a genuine respect for individual personality initiates a good relation between nurse and patient in the early settling in period and sustains it throughout the changes that must occur as the patient progresses towards complete recovery.

As the environment of hospital, its personnel and its routine become more familiar the first sharp anxieties aroused during the initial settling in period will have subsided and each patient will have adopted his own individual methods of coping with this big adjustment to such changed circumstances, the more usual of which we discussed in the previous chapter.

For all people who suffer a sharp break in their way of life such as is caused by coming into hospital there exists a considerable degree of anxiety regarding the human relationships and the responsibilities they have had temporarily to abandon.

The older school child or adolescent often worries about the time they are losing from school and from preparation for examinations which seem to matter vitally to the future course of their careers. Young people, new into jobs, may worry about holding their job if they are away from it too long. The young mother worries about her children. How are they being cared for? Are they fretting because she is away from them? How is her husband managing? For a husband there is the worry about being absent from his job or, in the case of serious illness, whether its effects will be so permanent that he will not be able to continue in the work to which he is accustomed. For most adults, coming into hospital involves leaving behind responsibilities and duties for which satisfactory arrangements cannot always be made. Patients long for news of home but quite frequently find it disturbing when they get it because it often discloses new problems about the family and work which they cannot deal with while in hospital and which merely instigate more anxiety.

According to his environmental circumstances, each patient has his own problems and worries. The nurse who sees her patient day by day and consequently builds up a very special relationship with him can frequently help to relieve anxiety simply by being willing to listen seriously and with interest to what the patient wishes to tell, regarding her patient's problems as part of her total picture of this sick person and a clue to her better understanding of him. She will of course also recognise the necessity of bringing this problem to the notice of those other members of the hospital staff whom it most concerns; for it is becoming increasingly recognised that recovery to total health after sickness depends on something much more than the medical treatment of the specific disease.

This can be seen most clearly in the changes and extensions of responsibility that have taken place in the work which now falls within the hospital almoner's field of duties. Almoners do much to help to sort out and alleviate the worries and problems in the patient's home life or work which illness is aggravating. Such services as provision of home help or arrangements for care of the children of a mother who is in hospital, the explanation to an employer of difficulties with regard to a patient's job arising from illness, arrangements for the rehabilitation of a person whose job has proved too exacting for him or for training for a new job in the case of a person whose illness has caused a disablement which rules out a return to his former type of work—all these fall within the responsibility of the almoner. She can be greatly helped in her work—as can also all the other members of the hospital staff concerned with the patient—by the nurse's sensitive awareness of her patient's needs, an awareness arising out of a relationship between nurse and patient built up through her day to day nursing care.

Perhaps the most difficult adjustments of all for an adult in hospital to make are those centring round the inevitable surrender of adult independence and of their right as an adult to make their own decisions and act on them. This revival of a condition of dependence inseparable from the nurse-patient relationship re-activates for most people many of the emotions relating to earlier phases of development. Those patients whose growth from the dependence of childhood was not achieved without emotional stress and difficulty often resist this new condition of dependence with a show of considerable resentment and antagonism towards the nurse. Others whose hold on the independence of maturity is still quite tenuous readily regress under the stress of their illness to a more childish pattern of behaviour and accept this new dependent situation wholly. In either case, the new relationship between patient and nurse resembles so closely patterns of behaviour relating to childhood that it is, as we saw in the previous chapter, difficult for many patients to keep their feelings towards the nurse entirely uncoloured by those that properly attached to people on whom they were emotionally dependent in childhood. As we saw earlier, this kind of projection of feeling takes place without the patient's conscious awareness. Nevertheless it may explain much in a patient's attitude and behaviour towards the nurse which would otherwise be puzzling in its inconsistency.

In the third or final stage of the illness, when the patient is beginning to move towards convalescence and recovery, there is a new shift of balance in the patient's relation to his nurse. The period of convalescence is often emotionally a very difficult one for the patient and consequently the progress towards complete recovery is usually an uneven one. All normal people want to be well again but recovery and the return to one's family and work and social community involves losing the attention, care, and freedom from responsibility that has characterised the period of sickness in hospital. Having again accepted and experienced some of the feeling of safety and reassurance that accompanied dependence, some people find it difficult to abandon it again and face the responsibilities and difficulties of life as an independent adult.

It is part of nursing skill to know how far to urge the patient to take over responsibility and do things for himself while avoiding pushing him too sharply towards independence when he still needs the emotional support of attention and care. It is during this period of convalescence that the therapeutic value of interests and occupation need to be recognised and exploited to the uttermost.

The nurse's task is fulfilled when her patient has not

only been nursed back to physical health but is also ready and able once more to face the responsibilities of life outside the hospital.

SUGGESTIONS FOR FURTHER READING

The First Five Years of Life. By A. Gesell and others. (Methuen).

The Nursery Years. By Susan Isaacs. (Routledge).

The Mothering of Young Children. By Gwendoline Chesters. (Faber & Faber).

The Natural Development of the Child. By Agatha Bowley. (Livingstone).

Infants without Families. By D. Burlingham and Anna Freud. (Allen & Unwin).

An Introduction to Child Guidance. By M. Burbury, E. Balint and B. Yapp. (Macmillan).

Girls Growing Up. By P. Jephcott (Faber & Faber).

General and Social Psychology. By R. H. Thouless. (University Tutorial Press).

Intelligence and Intelligence Testing. By Rex Knight. (Methuen).

Child Care and the Growth of Love. By J. Bowlby. (Pelican). A summary of the report prepared for the World Health Organisation. Abridged and edited by Margery Fry.

NOTE ON PSYCHOLOGICAL TERMS

IN writing this book I have tried wherever possible to avoid using technical terms and where this has been unavoidable have explained their meaning in the body of the text. One of the difficulties that is sometimes met with by beginners in the study of psychology arises from the fact that many terms which psychologists use with quite precise meaning are also in general usage in ordinary speech. Below are brief explanations therefore of a few of the terms likely to be met with in further reading and where the meaning that has become attached to them through popular usage may be misleading.

Students who want a more exhaustive dictionary are referred to: "A Dictionary of Psychology" by James Drever, published as a Penguin Reference Book, 2s. 6d.

Ability—what a person is able to do; his power to perform physical or mental acts in response to any stimulus or situation. The term *general ability* is used by psychologists to define the general mental power that is drawn on to some extent in the performance of every kind of task that we do and shows itself in every aspect of behaviour.

Affect—feelings or emotions which become attached to certain ideas. Thus the term *displacement of affect* is used to describe the shift of affect from the idea to which it properly belongs to a different idea. Or *fixation of affect* —a condition of mental development in which the individual remains attached to the feelings which rightly belong to an earlier phase of development.

Anxiety—a chronic and unresolved emotional attitude of fear, uncertainty and apprehension regarding the future.

Behaviour—the total response made by an individual to any situation with which he is faced.

Behaviourism—a term used to designate a theoretical approach to, or a "school" of psychological thought in which the main emphasis is placed on the objective study of "behaviour"; that is how a person reacts to any particular stimulus without any reference to conscious experience.

Emotion—a state of being which is accompanied by strong feeling and bodily changes such as, for example, in pulse rate, gland secretions etc., and which usually results in a characteristic form of behaviour dependent on the kind of emotion aroused.

Habit—an automatic way of reacting to certain specific situations which has been acquired by frequent repetition and learning. Organised habits of action and judgment by becoming automatic free a person from the need to give new attention and thought to his actions each time that particular set of circumstances arises. In this way his mental energy is freed for application to other tasks.

Instinct—a complex inherited tendency, usually accompanied by emotional excitement, which impels all individuals to act in a characteristic adaptive way apart from experience or learning. Instinct is the energy or drive which urges the individual to seek to attain a certain goal or purpose. Instinctive driving forces behind animal behaviour have have been grouped as follows: (i) instincts of self-preservation; (ii) instincts towards reproduction; (iii) social or gregarious instincts.

Psycho-analysis—a method of treating mental and nervous disorders based on the theoretical principles developed by Freud.

Psychiatrist—a medically qualified doctor who specialises in the treatment of disorders of the mind and of behaviour.

Psychology—the scientific study of the behaviour and experience of living organisms.

Psychologist—a person qualified in this study. The work of a psychologist may fall into several categories. An *academic psychologist* is normally engaged in teaching and research at a university. A psychologist who has qualified in the theory and science of psychology at a university may, however, have further training in applied psychology in one of various fields, for example as an *educational psychologist* trained in methods of applying the science of psychology to problems of education, an *industrial psychologist* trained in the application of psychology to human problems in industry and a *clinical psychologist* working in hospitals or pyschiatric clinics and trained to apply psychology to problems of mental illness and behaviour disorders.

Reflex action—an immediate muscular or glandular response to a sensory stimulus. It is an involuntary and unlearned response.

INDEX

For Product Safety Concerns and Information please contact our EU
representative GPSR@taylorandfrancis.com
Taylor & Francis Verlag GmbH, Kaufingerstraße 24, 80331 München, Germany

www.ingramcontent.com/pod-product-compliance
Ingram Content Group UK Ltd.
Pitfield, Milton Keynes, MK11 3LW, UK
UKHW022156190926
475702UK00003B/60
* 9 7 8 1 0 4 1 1 1 6 3 1 8 *